Pediatric Gastrointestinal Disorders

Pediatric Gastrointestinal Disorders

Biopsychosocial Assessment and Treatment

Carin L. Cunningham

Rainbow Babies and Children's Hospital
Case School of Medicine
Cleveland, Ohio

and

Gerard A. Banez

The Cleveland Clinic
Cleveland, Ohio

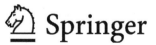

Carin L. Cunningham, Ph.D.
Department of Pediatrics
Division of Behavioral Pediatrics
Rainbow Babies and Children's
  Hospital
Case School of Medicine
Cleveland, Ohio 44106

Gerard A. Banez, Ph.D.
Division of Pediatrics/A120
The Cleveland Clinic Foundation
Cleveland, Ohio 44195

Cover illustration: Painting "Fantasy Intestines #4," © Seth Chwast Trust, photographed by Jane Critchlow and reproduced by permission of the artist.

Library of Congress Control Number: 2005924428

ISBN-10: 0-387-25611-3   e-ISBN 0-387-25612-1
ISBN-13: 978-0387-25611-5

Printed on acid-free paper.

Printed in the United States of America.   (SPI/EB)

9 8 7 6 5 4 3 2 1

springer.com

To the memory of Gerald Lamont (1912–2003), a wonderful father and supporter of my work

C. L. C.

Preface

As a postdoctoral fellow in pediatric psychology at a large tertiary medical center, Rainbow Babies and Children's Hospital, in Cleveland, Ohio, I was assigned to the pediatric gastroenterology clinic for a rotation. My responsibilities included direct patient care with pediatric and adolescent patients, consultation with pediatric gastroentrologists, and the planning and implementation of a group for parents of children and adolescents with inflammatory bowel disease (IBD). The collaboration was a positive experience for the physicians and myself.

I learned about the physical symptoms and the treatment of various gastrointestinal (GI) disorders that present in childhood and adolescents, a critical factor to ensure avoidance of the misattribution of psychological etiologies for physical symptoms. The pediatric gastroenterologists learned to identify behaviors that might be indicative of psychosocial issues.

When the three pediatric gastrolenterologists left that medical center for another hospital, they asked me to join their practice. For ten years I was a member of this practice whose strength was comprehensive, collaborative care provided to patients in a "user-friendly" manner. Thus, patients who might have been hesitant to consult a psychologist accepted the recommendation of the pediatric gastroenterologist, and the referral was presented in the context of a "team approach." Location in the same office was an added convenience, which facilitated the delivery of collaborative care. During that period, I evaluated and treated children and adolescents who presented with a finite number of medical diagnoses, but who also had a whole spectrum of psychological and behavioral issues. I provided behavioral intervention for toileting problems, psychotherapy for depressed adolescents dealing with complicated physical problems, and interventions for patients with pediatric feeding disorders. In addition to the direct patient care, I provided both formal and informal consultations with the gastroenterologists, which enhanced the care given, and frequently proved to be cost-effective in avoiding unnecessary hospitalizations or unnecessary medical follow-up visits.

I often saw patients who had seen other mental health professionals and who had attributed psychological causes to illness-related behaviors because they were not familiar with the specific GI symptoms or the treatment sequelae. I became aware that the mental health practitioner's knowledge, or lack of such, significantly impacted the treatment provided. For example, many of the presenting symptoms of IBD such as weight loss, fatigue, lack of energy, and abdominal pain were mistaken for depression or eating disorders by other mental health professionals. Children with severe constipation and subsequent stool withholding were thought to be "strong-willed, stubborn, and angry." These misconceptions often led to prolonging the problem and causing unnecessary guilt and shame for the child and the family. Our experience over a period of ten years was that collaborative treatment that included both physical and behavioral/psychological components resulted in successful outcomes for patients and their caregivers.

Ten years ago, the practice returned to Rainbow Babies and Children's Hospital, and I became an assistant professor in the Department of Pediatrics at Case Western Reserve School of Medicine. In addition to treating patients with GI disorders, I teach residents, behavioral pediatrician fellows, and psychology graduate students how behavioral and psychological factors interface with pediatric GI disorders. Four years ago, I began a toileting clinic for a wide range of children, which meets one morning a week. It has been very successful both as a clinical and teaching venue. My work has been intellectually challenging, and clinically satisfying.

Carin L. Cunningham

My initial exposure to the psychological assessment and treatment of pediatric GI problems came while I was a doctoral student in clinical psychology at the University of Vermont. During a clinical practicum in the Behavior Therapy and Psychotherapy Center, I was trained to provide biobehavioral treatments for one common GI disorder, fecal incontinence, and one less familiar disorder, aerophagia. These initial encounters kindled my interest in pediatric gastroenterology, raising my awareness of the importance of psychological/behavioral factors in understanding and treating these disorders. As a predoctoral intern and postdoctoral fellow at the Children's Hospital in Boston, I sought out additional experiences with pediatric GI problems. I learned more about the treatment of fecal incontinence, including the use of anorectal biofeedback to assist children with paradoxical contraction of the external anal sphincter. The level of functional disability experienced by these children can be significant, and the helping them maintain normal activity patterns, despite pain, became an emphasis in my clinical work.

My interest and involvement with GI problems continued in my first two positions after training. Though these positions did not allow me to specialize in the area, I continued to assess and treat children with recurrent abdominal pain and fecal incontinence. Upon my arrival at The Cleveland Clinic, I reimmersed myself in the field of pediatric gastroenterology. Shortly after starting my position, I became the primary psychology consultant to our Department of Pediatric GI and I began seeing a broader range of problems including rumination disorder, vomiting, irritable bowel syndrome, functional diarrhea, stool-toileting refusal, and inflammatory bowel disease. Currently, about one-half of my active caseload consists of patients referred by our pediatric gastroenterologists. My GI colleagues have been welcoming and supportive of my clinical services. Through our collaborative relationships, we have grown to recognize the importance of joint medical and psychological involvement for many children with GI problems. I am routinely consulted as part of the initial workup for children with recurrent abdominal pain (RAP) and frequently involved in the care of children with fecal incontinence and other GI symptoms. I see many of these children for management and follow-up. Over time, my involvement with our pediatric GI group has grown to include teaching of their trainees as well as multiple clinical research projects. As a psychologist, with my specialty interest, my role has been ideal and the collaborations have been fruitful and stimulating.

Gerard A. Banez

The purpose of this book is to provide relevant information and to share our clinical experience with the assessment and treatment of pediatric GI disorders. The book's specific objectives are:

1. To describe common pediatric gastrointestinal disorders and their psychological/behavioral correlates and sequelae.
2. To present conceptual/theoretical perspectives that guide understanding of etiology and treatment of these disorders.
3. To review empirically supported and clinically useful assessment and treatment strategies.
4. To be practice oriented but empirically informative (our overarching goal).

This book is intended as a reference guide and a manual for health care practitioners who work with children and adolescents with gastrointestinal disorders either from the medical perspective or the behavioral/mental health perspective. We have undertaken this project in an effort to share our knowledge and experience with the health care community. Our hope is that pediatric and adolescent patient care will continue to improve through the collaborative efforts of pediatricians, pediatric gastroenterologists, and their colleagues in psychology and behavioral medicine and that our experience working with these disorders will be useful to others.

Acknowledgments

I would like to acknowledge the help I have received from my pediatric colleagues in writing this book. My division chief, Dennis Drotar, Ph.D., has provided extensive support: introducing me to the pediatric GI team twenty years ago, supporting my professional endeavors as a faculty member over the past ten years, and, most recently, critiquing my chapters. Fred Rothstein, M.D., formerly the Chief of Pediatric Gastroenterology and presently the CEO of University Hospitals, had the vision twenty years ago to recognize that, in many cases, dealing exclusively with the child or adolescent's gastrointestinal tract was not the most effective treatment strategy. Consequently, he hired me as part of the PED GI practice that he and two other gastroenterologists created. It was in the PED GI practice that I learned specific information regarding the medical aspects of pediatric GI disorders and that I also had the opportunity to implement collaborative psychological and physical treatment modalities.

In addition to my aforementioned colleagues, I am indebted to Rosa Raskin, Director of the Pediatric Learning Center at Rainbow Babies and Children's Hospital. Her dedication and efficiency were invaluable in helping me to obtain information for this book. My coauthor, Gerard served as collaborator, support system, and friend throughout the process of writing this book. Dr. Samra Blanchard, a pediatric gastroenterologist at Rainbow Babies and Children's Hospital, helped me by reading the chapters and discussing relevant medical issues. Other pediatric colleagues whom I want to thank include: Jeffery Katz, M.D., Lara Bauman, MSN, Gisela Chelimsky, M.D., Kelly Wadeson, Ph.D., Daniel Cox, Ph.D., Steven Shapiro, M.D., Denise Bothe, M.D., Lynn Walker, Ph.D., and Melodie Sanders, B.A. My editors at Springer, Janice Stern and Herman Makler, were supportive and patient throughout this process. Steve Nipple's efforts were also essential in creating charts and typing many parts of the chapters that I wrote.

Finally I would like to thank my husband Michael for his patient support, his helpful advice, and his encouragement of my work over the past twenty years.

C.L.C.

Special thanks to Mariella, Chiara, Sophia, and Bianca, who shift my balance in the good and right direction. And to my parents, now Lolo and Lola, and sister, Carina, for their continuous love and support; Kokomo Joe, Nina, and all my out-laws; and my mentors, colleagues, and trainees, who have made the day-to-day rewarding and a lot of fun. And to Carin for asking me to write this book with her; and Herman and Janice. And especially to all the kids and families. They have always done the hard part.

G.A.B.

Contents

Biopsychosocial Factors That Impact
Pediatric Gastrointestinal Disorders

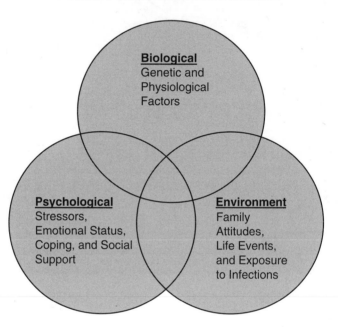

Pediatric Gastrointestinal Disorders: Prevalence, Costs, and Rationale for a Biopsychosocial Approach

IMPACT OF PEDIATRIC GASTROINTESTINAL DISORDERS

Gastrointestinal (GI) disorders in children are prevalent pediatric conditions that utilize significant health care resources (Guthery, Hutchings, Dean, & Hoff, 2004; Kugathasan et al., 2003). These disorders have a significant impact on a child's sense of physical and emotional well-being (Hyams, 2002; Loonen, Grootenhuis, Last, & Derkx, 2004; Voskuiji et al., 2004; Walker, 1999), and the ripple effects of these disorders extend to family members and caregivers. Pediatric gastrointestinal disorders can cause pain due to the symptoms of the disorder, the diagnostic testing, or the treatment modalities. Embarrassment due to symptoms such as repeated vomiting, fear of choking, excess flatulence, fecal soiling, the urgency to use the bathroom, or the sequelae of the disorder such as having an ostomy or episodes of fecal incontinence, is common and often traumatic for children, especially adolescents. School avoidance can become a chronic problem due to the hesitancy of using the toilets at school.

Children and adolescents are faced with the demands of normal development at the same time they are dealing with illness-related issues; consequently, normal developmental milestones may be affected. Physical sequelae such as delayed growth, inadequate nutritional status, and pain may persist even after treatment of the disorder (Hyams, 1996; Kirschner, 1990; Walker et al., 2001). Psychological development is impacted because these disorders interfere with normal developmental tasks such as independence with self-care, social relationships with peers, and the dynamics within the family (Engstrom & Lindquist, 1991; Mayberry, 1999; Moody, Eaden, & Mayberry, 1999). Body-image concerns due to the treatment of the disorders (e.g., having an ostomy) or to the medication side-effects (cushingoid features, weight gain, acne, mood swings from steroids for irritable bowel disease [IBD]) impact functioning with respect to peer relationships, school attendance, and the confidence to participate in age-appropriate activities (Banez & Cunningham, 2003; MacPhee, Hoffenberg, & Peranchak, 1988; Rabbett et al., 1996; Akobeng et al., 1999).

An issue unique to the management of pediatric GI disorders is that disorders such as irritable bowel syndrome (IBS) and recurrent abdominal pain (RAP) cause physical symptoms such as diarrhea, abdominal pain, or vomiting, yet the physical findings from diagnostic testing are not commensurate with the level of distress and pain reported by the child and the family. Some physicians, unable to document positive physical findings, automatically assume that the GI symptoms are caused by psychological factors, or may even doubt the validity of the disorders. Thus the child and the parents are frustrated and left to wonder if a physical disorder just has not yet been founded, or if the doctors just don't "believe" the child.

The following four cases illustrate the diverse range of problems seen in the field of pediatric gastroenterology. They also highlight the important role of psychological and behavioral factors in the etiology and treatment of GI disorders.

Abdominal Pain Case: Chelsea is a 9-year, 6-month-old fourth grader, who presents with a 2-year history of intermittent abdominal pain. She experiences little abdominal pain over school holidays and vacations, but has daily pain on school days. Chelsea's pain has significantly interfered with her daily functioning, particularly school attendance. She tends to keep her feelings to herself but often gets stressed or anxious at the onset of pain episodes. She identifies few personal coping strategies and is allowed to join her parents in bed when she has pain. Chelsea was diagnosed with gastroesophageal reflux and treated with multiple medications, but she continues to have pain.

Cyclic Vomiting Case: Ryan is a 7-year, 4-month-old second grader, who has bouts of severe nausea and vomiting that usually last 1 to 4 days, separated by symptom-free intervals. He averages as many as 9 to 12 vomiting episodes per year. Numerous medical explanations for his vomiting have been ruled out, so the causes for his vomiting are not clear. Though medications are occasionally effective in aborting vomiting at onset, little is helpful once the episode begins.

Fecal Incontinence: Jake is a typically developing 4-year-old boy who is having difficulty mastering toilet training with respect to his bowel movements. He withholds his stool stating that he is afraid "that it will hurt." He is resistant to using the toilet for stooling, preferring to stool in a corner of his bedroom. His parents have tried many approaches including rewards and punishment without achieving any success or even progress. They have become increasingly frustrated. Jake's pediatrician tells his parents not to pressure him and that he "will do it when he's ready."

Inflammatory Bowel Disease: Beth is a 16-year-old girl with Crohn's disease, diagnosed when she was 10 years old. The course of her illness has been variable. She was initially placed on a course of a high dose of steroids, which caused significant side effects including: weight gain, cushingoid features, and acne. She improved and the steroids were decreased, and then stopped. Recently, Beth has had a flare-up of her Crohn's disease and the steroid medication was restarted. Beth has become increasingly depressed especially with the return of the side effects. Her parents have found pills that she has hidden and arguments over noncompliance have increased significantly.

These cases illustrate that pediatric GI disorders are typically the result of a combination of psychosocial factors in addition to physical symptoms. The configuration of how physical symptoms and psychosocial factors interact is unique to each patient. As Drossman states, "It is no longer rational to try to discriminate whether physiological or psychologic factors cause pain or other bowel symptoms. Both are operative, and the task is to determine the degree to which each contributes and is remediable" (Drossman et al., 1999, pp. II26). Thus the treatment of pediatric GI disorders presents new challenges with each patient.

In this chapter, we begin by examining the prevalence data for the pediatric Gl disorders. The costs of these disorders, both monetary expense and the potential impact on functioning, are examined. A rationale for the biopsychosocial approach for the treatment of pediatric GI disorders is presented in Table 1.1. As can be seen from the data in Table 1.1, six disorders (inflammatory bowel disease, esophageal disorders, vomiting disorders, recurrent abdominal pain [RAP], irritable bowel syndrome [IBS], and fecal incontinence [FI]) affect a significant number of children and adolescents. Three common pediatric GI disorders—IBS, RAP, and GER—each affect about 10% or more of the pediatric population. Recent epidemiological studies report that the incidence of Crohn's disease is increasing in the pediatric population (Kugathasan et al., 2003), while for other disorders such as globus sensation and rumination disorders no pediatric data are available as of yet.

COSTS OF GASTROINTESTINAL DISORDERS: IMPACT ON FUNCTIONING AND ECONOMIC COSTS

National estimates of the burden of pediatric GI disorders as a whole are largely underreported. The paucity of data may be due to the following factors: (1) the inclusion of children in adult studies of GI disorders, (2) the focus on more common pediatric conditions such as asthma, and (3) the lack of datasets with information on pediatric GI disorders (Guthery et al., 2004).

The Kids' Inpatient Database (KID) is a special subset of the health care cost and utilization project, which enables analyses of hospital utilization by children across the United States. Data from KID indicates that the most common GI disorders in hospitalized children are acute diarrheal diseases, appendicitis, abdominal pain, esophageal disorders, and digestive congenital anomalies. This small number of diagnoses accounts for 75.1% of all GI discharge diagnoses, 64.2% of all GI hospital charges, and 68% of all GI hospital days. Data for actual costs are available from pediatric discharge

TABLE 1.1. Prevalence of Pediatric Gastrointestinal Disorders

Gastrointestinal Disorder	Prevalence	Reference
1. **Inflammatory Bowel Disease (Pediatrics)**	30% of all patients with IBD	Pappa et al., 2004
a. Crohn's disease	a. 4.56/100,000	a. Kugathasan et al., 2003
b. Ulcerative colitis	b. 2.14/100,000	b. Kugathasan et al., 2003
c. Indeterminate colitis	c. 15% of cases of IBD	c. King, 2003
2. **Esophageal Disorders**		
a. Globus sensation	a. No data available in children	
b. Infant with recurrent regurgitation	b. Daily regurgitation in 50% of infants 2-8 mos, 66% of infants < 4 mos, 5% of infants < 1 year	b. Vanderplas et al., 2002; Orenstein et al., 1999
c. GERD	c. Heartburn: 1.8%: 3-9 y/o, 3.5% adolescents	c. Orenstein et al., 1999
d. NEMD's	d. Regurgitation: 2.3% 3-9 y/o, 1.4% adolescents	d. Rosario et al., 1999
3. **Vomiting Disorders**		
a. Rumination	a. Uncommon, no recent prevalence reports	a. Singh, 1981; Whitehead, 1985; Schuster, 1985
b. Cyclic vomiting	b. 2%	b. Forbes et al., 1999
4. **Recurrent Abdominal** Pain (RAP)	9-25% of all children	Apley & Nash, 1958;
	a. 10-15% school age	a. Oster, 1972; Apley, 1975
	b. Almost 20% middle h.s.	b. Hyams et al., 1996
5. **Irritable Bowel** Syndrome (IBS)	a. 6% middle school	Hyams, 1996
	b. 14% high school	
6. **Fecal Incontinence (FI)**	1-3% pediatric population	Fishman et al., 2003
a. Retentive (RFI)	a. 80-95% of children with FI	a. Loening-Bauche, 1993
b. Non-retentive (NRFI)	b. 10-20% of children with FI	b. Taubman, 1997

data in 1997 when there were 329,825 pediatric discharges associated with a principal GI diagnosis, which represents 9.1% of all discharges, 7.9% of all total charges, and 7.4% of all hospital days, excluding delivery of newborns.

These admissions accounted for $2.6 billion and 1.1 million hospital days. The mean and median hospital charge per hospitalization of children with a GI discharge diagnosis was $8,155 and $4,441, respectively (Guthery et al., 2004). For pediatric patients with functional gastrointestinal disorders (FGIDs), additional costs may be those associated with tests that are done to exclude medical diagnoses.

Epidemiological studies report that the U.S. Public Health Service has underestimated the prevalence of FGIDs, which includes RAP and IBS (Locke, 1996). Underestimation is attributed to the fact that subjects were asked to report diagnoses rather than specific symptoms and that current medical coding did not provide specific codes for each of the FGIDs. Table 1.2

TABLE 1.2. Potential Impact on Functioning and Costs of GI Disorders in Children and Adolescents

GI Disorder	Potential Impact on Functioning	Monetary Cost
Cyclic Vomiting	1. Despite the fact that children with CV are ill less than 10% of time, there is substantial academic and medical morbidity 2. The mean number of school absences was 24 days/year 3. The rate of IV hydration was 58% of patients seen (Li Buk, Misiewicz, 2003)	The average annualized cost of ER visits, hospital stays, and testing was $17,035/pt. (Li Bu & Misiewicz, 2003)
Fecal Incontinence	1. Children with FI represent 25-30% of patients seen in a pediatric GI practice and 1-3% of pediatric outpatient visits (Loening-Baucke, 1999) 2. Psychosocial sequelae for untreated FI can include social isolation, family conflicts and school avoidance 3. Young children with FI cannot attend preschool 4. Parents experience pressure from family members and doubt their parenting skills	1. Cost of Miralax is $40/bottle which typically lasts for a month 2. Costs diapers/pull-ups increase environmental waste nonbiodegradable 3. Inpatient cost of golytely clean-out approximately $1,000 4. Costs of follow-up appointments and X-rays
Inflammatory Bowel Disease	1. Peak age of onset of IBD is between 15-25 years of age (Kugathasan, 2003) 2. Approximately 25% of all new cases of Crohn's disease and between 15% and 40% of new cases of ulcerative colitis are diagnosed in individuals younger than 20 years of age 3. Half to three-fourths of children with CD eventually require surgery because of not responding to medical therapy (Kay & Wyllie 2003) 4. Patients limit their functioning in extracurricular activities due to fatigue 5. There is an increase in anxiety due to the uncertainty of the course of the illness 6. Growth and development is often delayed (Kirschner, 1990)	1. Average annual charges for CD pts. $12,417 (Feagan et al., 2000) 2. Remicade (Inflixamab) infusions cost approximately $2,000/pt. leave infusions 3. Costs, procedures, medications surgeries, F/U visits

Continued

TABLE 1.2. (cont.)

Irritable Bowel Syndrome	1. IBS is the second most common cause of work and school related absenteeism 2. IBS-like symptoms were present in the majority of children presenting to a pediatric gastroenterology clinic with recurrent abdominal pain 3. School avoidance can become a chronic problem because of early morning cramping and dislike of using school restrooms	1. Total costs of care were 49% higher than age/sex-matched controls. 2. Total costs of health care through insurance plan in oneyear $4,376. (Levy et al., 2001) 3. IBS direct and indirect costs > $30 billion/year (Hyams, 1996)
Esophageal Disorders	1. Potential negative impact of caregiver/child relationship (GER) 2. Anxiety over eating in front of others leading to isolation, weight loss (globus) 3. Abdominal pain complaints due to chronic reflux (GERD) 4. Undetected anxiety disorders that can co-occur with physical problems	1. 10% of all pediatric hospital admissions in U.S. and Canada are related to GERD 2. 1997 U.S. hospital data: 77,560 patients > 17 y/age diagnosed with GERD 3. Mean hospital stay of 3.9-5.7 days; mean Charge $7,032 to $13, 507 per patient (Czinn et al., 2002)
Recurrent Abdominal Pain	1. Adoption of "sick role" identity 2. School absences leading to avoidance 3. Isolation from friends because of lack or participation in age appropriate activities 4. Frustration because of the lack of medical diagnosis to explain pain	1. Costs of unnecessary tests 2. Costs of unneeded hospitalizations and doctor visits 3. Costs of medications both over the counter and prescribed

presents the costs of pediatric GI disorders with respect to both the potential impact on functioning and the monetary costs associated with these disorders. Table 1.2 is a descriptive listing of the potential psychological burden of pediatric GI disorders and the practical costs of care. Increasingly, there is awareness that management of GI conditions should include measures of patient's health-related quality of life (HRQOL), which encompasses the physical, social, and emotional effect of health disorders. HRQOL is increasingly being used as a treatment outcome measure in evaluating the impact in a range of pediatric GI disorders (Yousseff, 2004). Studies using both a generic instrument and a disease-specific measure have demonstrated that the HRQOL of children and adolescents with IBD is impaired in comparison to healthy controls (Loonen et al., 2004; Pace et al., 2003; Cunningham, Drotar, Palermo,

McGowan, & Arendt, 2006). A new disease-specific instrument to measure the impact of defecation disorders has been constructed (Voskuiji et al., 2004). Studies of patients with IBS have demonstrated that they experience psychological distress and a diminished HRQOL (Bulavari & Olden, 2004; Drossman, 1998; Whitehead, Burnett, Cook, & Taub, 1996).

In addition to the potential impact on functioning for the child and the financial costs of medical care, significant stress is placed on the patient's family or caregiver of a child with a GI disorder, since in pediatric care, the patient is not just the child but also the child-parent unit (Drotar, 1981; Hyams, 1996). Our clinical experience indicates that pediatric GI disorders affect the child and the family and that there is a reciprocal aspect: often children can be affected by their parents' worries about them. Parents have reported the following concerns:

1. They worry about the impact of their child's GI disorder: Will development proceed in a typical manner? Will their child adopt a "sick" role identity?
2. Parents have concerns about their child's peer relationships: Will they be teased because of their having to use the bathroom excessively, or because of embarrassing bodily sounds or smells, or physical changes due to medication side effects?
3. Parents question if the disorders have long-term psychological consequences: Will the child internalize shame or a poor body image because of these symptoms?
4. Many parents question, "Did we do something wrong?" even in light of positive physical findings. If the physical findings are unremarkable, parents question if the doctors have "missed something."
5. School attendance is a concern, whether it is preschool for parents of children with fecal incontinence or college for adolescents with IBD.

Clinicians working with children and adolescents have the opportunity to mitigate the psychosocial costs of pediatric GI disorders for children and their caregivers, and to maximize their developmental course despite the significant physical and psychological demands of these disorders.

RATIONALE FOR A BIOPSYCHOSOCIAL APPROACH TO PEDIATRIC GI DISORDERS

Three issues underscore the importance of a biopsychosocial perspective in evaluating and treating pediatric gastrointestinal disorders. The first is that psychological and environmental factors impact the etiology and the course of many GI disorders (Drossman, 1998; Lackner, Mesmer, Morley, Dowzer, & Hamilton, 2004; Loonen et al., 2004; Walker, 1999). Consequently, for treatment to be effective these factors must be addressed (Whitehead & Schuster, 1985). Increasingly, evidence-based research is reporting that biomedical treatments of GI disorders that ignore psychological and behavioral contributions are not as effective as a biopsychosocial approach (Finney, Lemanek, Cataldo, Katz, & Fuqua, 1989; Lackner et al., 2004; McGrath, Mellon, & Murphy, 2000; Richter & Bradley, 1996; Sanders et al., 1989).

The second issue that supports a biopsychosocial perspective is the awareness that the clinician is treating a dynamic process: the developing child or adolescent and not just their GI tract. A biopsychosocial approach can enhance treatment and potentially avoid further sequelae. For example, in adolescents, the potential impact of physical changes due to medication side effects of steroid treatment for Crohn's disease (CD) may lead to problems with noncompliance. Anticipatory guidance regarding this issue may aid in avoiding or lessening future problems. Likewise, awareness of issues of independence and developing autonomy in a 4-year-old child with retentive fecal incontinence is important in the process of creating and implementing a behavioral treatment plan. The child who actively participates in choosing the components of their behavioral modification plan (e.g., the specific times for practice sits, the rewards and consequences when goals are not met) is more likely in our experience to cooperate with the plan and to be more successful. In general, treatment that recognizes developmental issues will benefit from the forward propulsion that growth and development provide.

The third issue that supports a biopsychosocial approach is the potential cost offset that the addition of psychosocial interventions can bring to the care of children with GI disorders. Public health care systems and third-party payers are increasingly using economic theory to consider resource allocation problems in health care and to provide evidence of the relative cost-effectiveness of different drugs, diagnostic and therapeutic interventions, and health services in order to aid prioritization (Edwards & Thalanany, 2001). The ability of psychological interventions to reduce general medical costs has been termed the "medical cost–offset effect" by Chiles, Lambert, and Hatch (1999), which is used to determine the efficacy of various psychosocial interventions in treating children with medical issues.

A meta-analysis of 91 studies to evaluate the impact of psychological interventions on the use of medical services provided evidence for a medical cost–offset effect (Chiles et al., 1999). The most dramatic treatment effects were demonstrated in the use of behavioral medicine techniques to treat surgical inpatients, which led to a significant decrease in length of stay for surgical patients and an increase in psychological well-being. Savings of approximately 20% from implementing psychological interventions were noted, even when the costs of those interventions were subtracted from the savings. Although few in number, studies of children suggest a larger offset than persons aged 18 to 64. Children who overutilize medical services appear to decrease their physician visits when provided psychoeducational training and psychotherapy (Finney, Riley, & Cataldo, 1991).

Depressed mood, persistent anxiety, and related impaired function are associated with substantial increases in the use and cost of general medical care (Hunkeler, Spector, Fireman, Rice, & Weisner, 2003). The effects are additive: the more psychological problems that exist, the greater the increase in medical care costs. Yet, pathways that define this linkage are unclear and poorly defined. Persistent anxiety may increase health care costs because of altered self-assessments of health: children with IBS may have heightened sensitivity to their intestinal motility. Their responses to these subtle physical cues or sensations may be interpreted as pain, which can impact coping responses including health care–seeking behavior. The effects of reducing anxiety on health care utilization remain unknown, as are the effects of reducing anxiety in parents of children with GI disorders or symptoms.

Clinical experience provides many specific examples where psychosocial intervention directly impacted a decrease in medical health costs. The following three examples come from the first author's experience over the past 20 years.

Children with retentive fecal incontinence (RFI) who are treated with only medical management have more inpatient hospitalizations for golytely cleanouts, more follow-up appointments with pediatric gastroenterologists, and more problems with noncompliance in comparison to children who are treated with a comprehensive approach, including education and a behavioral modification program. Anecdotal experience is consistent with the evidence-based data that report medical management combined with behavioral modification training is more effective and results in better outcomes for children with RFI (McGrath et al., 2000).

Although RAP is not necessarily indicative of a psychopathology, patterns of secondary gain or avoidance of issues at school may be unknowingly contributing to the maintenance of this problem. Our experience has been that managing patients with RAP in a comprehensive manner can avoid unnecessary costs associated with expensive diagnostic tests, repeat hospitalizations and emergency room visits, as well as unnecessary physician appointments.

Children who present with the globus sensation, fear of choking because "something is stuck," but with no positive physical findings, can potentially be at risk for eating problems, which if not treated can lead to weight loss and nutritional deficits. Education and reassurance of the child and parents coupled with behavioral management has in our experience been very effective: most children return to eating solid food. A decrease in anxiety about the globus sensation can avoid further invasive testing, and that energy can be redirected to dealing with the treatment plan.

Finally, an additional factor in decreasing costs is the impact that anxious caregivers or parents have on the maintenance of their child's symptoms and on the health care–seeking behavior. This can be seen in mothers of infants with age-appropriate GER, with parents who are embarrassed or anxiously focused on toilet training issues, or with parents of children with RAP who are convinced that despite normal physical findings, a physical problem is the etiology of their child's complaints. These caregivers may pressure physicians for further diagnostic tests or treatments because of their own level of high anxiety.

As yet there are no published data documenting the cost savings of a biopsychosocial approach to the treatment of pediatric GI disorders, despite the fact that our clinical experiences are replete with such examples across the array of pediatric GI disorders that will be discussed in this book.

SUMMARY

This chapter documents that pediatric gastrointestinal disorders are common in children and adolescents. They cause physical discomfort, emotional anguish, and they can affect development. The monetary costs are high due to the need for special medical procedures, diagnostic tests, medication, and office visits. Our experience provides anecdotal confirmation for the positive effects resulting from assessing and treating pediatric GI disorders from a biopsychosocial perspective. A cost-offset trend is indicated in treating children with behavioral interventions to reduce costs associated with medical treatment.

REFERENCES

Akobeng, A. K., Suresh-Babu, M. V., Firth, D., Miller, V., Mir, P., & Thomas, A. G. (1999). Quality of life in children with Crohn's disease: a pilot study. *Journal of Pediatric Gastroenterology Nutrition, 4*, S37–39.

Apley, J. (1975). *The child with abdominal pain* (2nd ed.). London: Blackwell.

Apley, J., & Nash, N. (1958). Recurrent abdominal pain: A field survey of 1000 school children. *Archives of Diseases of Childhood, 33*, 165–170.

Banez, G., & Cunningham, C. (2003). Pediatric gastrointestinal disorders: Recurrent abdominal pain, inflammatory bowel disease, and rumination disorder/cyclic vomiting. In M. C. Roberts (Ed.), *Handbook of pediatric psychology* (pp. 462–478). New York: Guilford.

Chiles, J., Lambert, M. J., & Hatch, A. L. (1999). The impact of psychological interventions on medical cost offset: A meta-analytic review. *Clinical Psychology: Science and Practice, 6*(2).

Cunningham, C., Drotar, D., Palermo, T., McGowan, K., Arendt, R. (2006). Health-related quality of life in children and adolescents with inflammatory bowel disease. *Submitted manuscript.*

Czinn, S., Gold, B., Dickinson, C., Ramakrishna, J., & Orenstein, S. (2002). Research agenda for pediatric gastroenterology, hepatology and nutrition: Acid-peptic diseases. *Journal of Pediatric Gastroenterology Nutrition, 35*(3), 250–253.

Drossman, D. A. (1998). Presidential address: Gastrointestinal illness and the biopsychosocial model. *Pyschosomatic Medicine, 60*(3), 258–267.

Drossman, D. A., Creed, F. H., Olden, K. W., Svedlund, J., Toner, B. B., Whitehead, W. E. (1999). Psychosocial aspects of the functional gastrointestinal disorders. *Gut, 45* Suppl 2:II25–II30.

Drotar, D. (1981). Psychological perspectives in chronic childhood illness. *Journal of Pediatric Psychology, 6*(3), 211–228.

Edwards, R. T., & Thalanany, M. (2001). Trade-offs in the conduct of economic evaluations of child mental health services. *Mental Health Services Research, 3*(2), 99–105.

Engstrom, I., & Lindquist, B. L. (1991). Inflammatory bowel disease in children and adolescents: A somatic and psychiatric investigation. *Acta Paediatrica Scandavica, 80*, 640–647.

Feagan, B. G., Vreeland, M. G., Larson, L., Bala, M. V. (2000). Annual cost of care for crohn's disease: A payor perspective. *American Journal of Gastroenterology, 95*(2), 1955–1960.

Finney, J. W., Riley, A. W., Cataldo, M. F. (1991). Psychology in primary healthcare: Effects of brief targeted therapy on children's medical care utilization. *Journal of Pediatric Psychology, 16*(4), 447–461.

Finney, J. W., Lemanek, K. L., Cataldo, M. F., Katz, H. P., & Fuqua, R. W. (1989). Pediatric psychology in primary health care: Brief targeted therapy for recurrent abdominal pain. *Behavior Therapy, 20*, 283–291.

Fishman, L., Rappaport, L., Schonwald, A., & Nurko, S. (2003). Trends in referral to a single encopresis clinic over 20 years. *Pediatrics, 111*(5), 604–607.

Forbes, D., Withers, G., Silburn, S., & McKelvey, R. (1999, August). Psychological and social characteristics and precipitants of vomiting in children with Cyclic vomiting syndrome. *Digestive Diseases and Sciences, 8*(Suppl.), S19–S22.

Guthery, S. L., Hutchings, C., Dean, J. M., & Hoff, C. (2004). National estimates of hospital utilization by children with gastrointestinal disorders: analysis of the 1997 KIDs' inpatient database. *Journal of Pediatrics, 144*, 589–594.

Hunkeler, E. M., Spector, W. D., Fireman, B., Rice, D. P., & Weisner, C. (2003, May–June). Psychiatric symptoms, impaired function, and medical care costs in an HMO setting. *General Hospital Psychiatry, 25*(3), 178–184.

Hyams, J. S. (1999). Chronic and recurrent abdominal pain. In P.E. Hyman (Ed.), *Pediatric functional gastrointestinal disorders* (pp. 7.1–7.21). New York: Academic Professional Information Services.

Hyams, J. S. (2002). *Pediatric functional gastrointestinal disorders.* New York: Academy Professional Information Services.

Kay, M., & Wyllie, R. (2003, April). The real cost of pediatric Crohn's disease: The role of inliximab in the treatment of pediatric IBD. *American Journal of Gastroenterology, 98*(4), 712–720.

King, R. A. (2003). Pediatric inflammatory bowel disease. *Child Adolescent Psychiatric Clinics of North America, 12*(3), 537–550.

Kirschner, B. S. (1990). Growth and development in chronic inflammatory bowel disease. *Acta Paediatrica Scandinavica, 366*(Suppl.), 98–104.

Kugathasan, S., Judd, R. H., Hoffman, R. G., Heikenen, J., Telega, G., Khan, F. et al. (2003). (2003). Epidemiologic and clinical characteristics of children with newly diagnosed inflammatory bowel disease in Wisconsin: A statewide population-based study. *Journal of Pediatrics, 143*, 525–531.

Lackner, J. M., Mesmer, C., Morley, S., Dowzer, C., & Hamilton, S. (2004). Psychological treatments for irritable bowel syndrome: A systematic review and meta-analysis. *Journal of Consulting and Clinical Psychology, 72*(6), 1100–1113.

Levy, R. L., Von Korff, M., Whitehead, W., Stang, W. E., Saunders, K., Jhingram, P. et al. (2001). Costs of care for irritable bowel syndrome patients in a health V, maintenance organization. *American Journal of Gastroenterology, 96*, 3122–3129.

Li Bu, Misiewicz (2003). Cyclic vomiting syndrome: A brain–got disorder. *Gastroenterology Clinics of North America, 32*(3), 997–1019.

Locke, R. G. (1996). Epidemiology of functional gastrointestinal disorders in North America. *Gastroenterology Clinics of North America, 25*(1), 1–19.

Loening-Baucke, V. (1993). Constipation in early childhood: Patient characteristics, treatment and long-term follow-up. *Gut, 34*, 1400–1404.

Loonen, H. J., Grootenhuis, M. A., Last, B. F., & Derkx, H. H. F. (2004). Coping strategies and quality of life of adolescents with inflammatory bowel disease. *Quality of Life Research, 13*, 1011–1019.

MacPhee, M., Hoffenberg, E. J., & Peranchak, A. (1988). Coping strategies and quality of life factors in adolescents with inflammatory bowel disease. *Inflammatory Bowel Disorder, 1*, 6–11.

Mayberry, J. F. (1999). Impact of inflammatory bowel disease on educational achievements and work prospects. *Journal of Pediatric Gastroenterology and Nutrition, 28*, S34–S36.

McGrath, M. L., Mellon, M. W., & Murphy, L. (2000). Empirically supported treatment in pediatric psychology: Constipation and encopresis. *Journal of Pediatric Psychology, 25*, 225–254.

Moody, G., Eaden, J., & Mayberry, J. (1999). Social implications of childhood Crohn's disease. *Journal of Pediatric Gastroeneterology and Nutrition, 28*, S43–S45.

Orenstein, S. R., Izadnia, F., & Khan, S. (1999). Gastroesophageal reflux disease in children. In G. E. Katz (Ed.), *Gastroenterology clinics of North America* (pp. 947–969). Philadelphia: W. B. Saunders.

Oster, J. (1972). Recurrent abdominal pain, headache and limb pains in children and adolescents. *Pediatrics, 50*, 429–436.

Pace, F., Molteni, P., Bollani, S., Sarzi-Puttini, P., Stockbrugger, R., Bianchi Porro, G., & Drossman, D. A. (2003). Inflammatory bowel disease versus irritable bowel syndrome: A hospital based, case-control study of disease impact on quality of life. *Scandinavian Journal of Gastroenterology, 38*(10), 1031–1038.

Pappa, H. M., Semrin, G., Walker, T. R., & Grand, R. J. (2004). Pediatric inflammatory bowel disease. *Current Opinion in Gastroenterology, 20*, 333–340.

Rabbett, H., Elbadri, A., Thwaites, R., Northover, H., Dady, I., Firth, D., Hillier, V. F., Miller, V., Thomas, A. G. (1996). Quality of life in children with Crohn's disease. *Journal of Pediatric Gastroenterology and Nutrition, 23*(5), 528–533.

Rather, L. J. (1965). *Mind and body in eighteenth century medicine: A study based on Jerome Gaub De-Regime-mentis.* Berkeley: University of California Press.

Richter, J. E., & Bradley, L. C. (1996, October). Psychophysiological interactions in esophageal diseases. *Seminars in Gastrointestinal Disease, 7*(4), 169–184.

Rosario, J. A., Medow, M. S., Halata, M. S., Bostwick, H. E., Newman, L. J., Schwarz, S. M. et al. (1999, May). Nonspecific esophageal motility disorders in children without gastro-esophageal reflux. *Journal of Pediatric Gastroenterology Nutrition, 28*(5), 480–485.

Sander, M. R., Rebgetz, M., Morrison, M., Bor, W., Gordon, A., Dadds, M. et al. (1989). Cognitive-behavioral treatment of recurrent non-specific abdominal pain in children: An analysis of generalization, maintenance, and side-effects. *Journal of Consulting and Clinical Psychology, 57*, 294–300.

Singh, N. N. (1981). Rumination. In N. R. Ellis (Ed.), *International review of research in mental retardation* (p. 10). New York: Academic Press.

Talley, N. J., Gabriel, S. E., Harmsen, W. S., Zinsomeister, A. R., & Evans, R. W. (1995). Medical costs in community subjects with irritable bowel syndrome. *Gastroenterology, 109*, 1736–1741.

Taubman, B. (1997). Toilet training and toileting refusal for stool only: A prospective study. *Pediatrics, 99*, 54–58.

Vandenplas, Y., & Hassall, E. (2002). Mechanisms of gastroesophageal reflux and gastro-esophageal reflux disease. *Journal of Pediatric Disease and Nutrition, 35*, 119–136.

Voskuijl, W. P., van der Zaag-Loonen, H. J., Ketel, I. J. G., Grootenhuis, M. A., Derkx, B. H. B., & Benning, M. A. (2004). Health related quality of life in disorders of defecation: The defecation disorder list. *Archives of Disease in Childhood, 89*, 1124–1127.

Walker, L. S. (1999, October). Pathways between recurrent abdominal pain and adult functional gastrointestinal disorders. *Journal of Developmental and Behavioral Pediatrics, 20*(5), 320–322.

Whitehead, W. E., Burnett, C. K., Cook, E. W., III, & Taub, E. (1996). Impact of irritable bowel syndrome on quality of life. *Digestive Diseases and Sciences, 41*, 2248–2253.

Whitehead, W. E., & Schuster, M. M. (1985). Rumination syndrome, vomiting aerophagia, and belching. In W. E. Whitehead & M. M. Schuster (Eds.), *Gastrointestinal disorders: Behavioral and physiological basis for treatment* (pp. 67–90). Orlando, FL: Academic Press.

Youssef, N. (2004). IBD or IBS: When there is abdominal pain, does it really matter? *Journal of Pediatric Gastroenterology and Nutrition, 38*, 460–461.

Theoretical and Historical Basis for a Biopsychosocial Approach to Pediatric Gastrointestinal Disorders

2

This chapter provides a historical and theoretical context for a biopsychosocial approach to the pediatric gastrointestinal (GI) disorders. The discussion follows a progression from general mind/body issues to the specific relationship between mind/body issues in pediatric GI disorders. Then pediatric functional GI disorders are examined. Finally, the basis for pediatric GI disorders from a brain–gut axis perspective is discussed.

HISTORICAL REVIEW OF MIND/BODY RELATIONSHIP

The relationship between the mind, "psyche," and the body, "soma," in the causation and treatment of physical problems has a complex history in Western medicine that has yet to be satisfactorily resolved in contemporary times. Aristotle in the 4th century B.C. stated, "The body and the soul or psyche are reciprocally connected through the individual's temperament and consequently influence each other"; separation between them does not exist (Roccatagliata, 1997).

In medieval times, the mind/body dilemma was viewed as a religious issue, and the Catholic Church institutionalized the theory of a separation of the body and the soul. The mind and the "transfer of the soul" were under the purview of the church; the body was seen as an imperfect ("sinful") organ, a viewpoint that sanctioned the dissection of the human body. Descartes in the early 1600s proposed a model that identified differences between the mind, "res. Cognate," a thing, which thinks, and the body, "res. Extensa," which could be measured because it occupies space. Descartes's theory of dualism conceptualized the human body as mechanistic and reducible to elementary parts and systems. The scientific approach to disease at this time further reinforced the notion that the body was a machine; disease was the malfunctioning of the machine. The impact of behavioral and psychosocial processes was ignored (Drossman, 1998).

During the 18th and 19th centuries the mind/body dilemma swung back and forth between an integrated concept and a dualist concept, with dualism

13

remaining the driving force and the dominant view. The discovery of microorganisms by Pasteur and Koch's development of the *germ theory* of disease propelled medicine toward a biomedical model (Ray, 2004). Little connection was seen between the mind and the body; illness was viewed as the result of organic pathology.

In the 20th century the issue of psychosocial versus biological influences regarding the etiology of physical problems cycled even more rapidly. In the 1920s, Flanders Dunbar (1954) introduced the term psychosomatic, which she defined as, "physical disorders, which are caused by or exacerbated by psychological factors," with the autonomic nervous system serving as the mediator between emotions and the physical responses of the body. Phenomena were observed concurrently from somatic and psychic angles, and studies examined physiological changes accompanying emotion.

Psychiatry, influenced by Freudian theory, continued to study the psychological aspects of general and specific medical problems. However, the mediator between emotions and physical illnesses was transformed into a symbolic one: unresolved dynamic emotional conflicts were associated with and thought to cause selected physical disorders such as asthma, ulcerative colitis, and peptic ulcer disease. Patients with ulcerative colitis were described as "passive, emotionally immature and pathologically attached to their mother" (Murray-Lyon & Perkin, 1998, p. 292), while children with fecal incontinence were described as "using soiling as a means of gaining attention within the context of a hostile dependency relationship with their mother" (Ringdahl, 1980, p. 65). Evidence from case reports based on descriptive observational information and correlation data was used to support the relationship between stressful life events, personality profiles, and specific organ dysfunctions or illnesses. Despite the initial wide acceptance of this theory, to date, there has been no scientific evidence that emotions "pile up" and that unresolved psychological conflicts are converted to somatic symptoms or diseases (Wilhelmsen, 2000).

In the 1960s biomedical research resulted in significant advances in the treatment of physical illnesses. The biomedical model, which originated with Pasteur, became prominent. In the biomedical model, disease is accounted for by deviations from the norm of measurable biological (somatic) variables: all biological phenomena can be explained by chemistry and physics. Disease is seen as independent of social behavior or psychological functioning, and behavioral differences are the result of disordered biochemical or neurophysiological processes and categorized as mental diseases (Ray, 2004; Entralgo, 1956).

The psychosomatic model and the biomedical model both have limitations: they are unidirectional models that are unable to account for the complex interaction of factors that impact an individual's functioning and the variety of idiosyncratic responses to physical symptoms. Neither model explains why some people with positive physical findings report feeling well, while others whose physical tests produce normal results complain of severe pain. Although about 40% to 60% of the population has Helicobacter pylori, the most common cause of peptic ulcer disease (PUD) in their GI lining, only 7% of the individuals with Helicobacter pylori develop ulcer disease. Depression and life stressors, which increase gastric acid secretion, may increase an individual's risk. However, for some patients with PUD, emotional factors are irrelevant (Levenstein, 2000). How do we account for the variability of response to Helicobacter pylori?

In 1977 Engel proposed the biopsychosocial model that encompasses physical, psychological, and environmental factors and reconciles the complicated interactions and pathways among them that can lead to a disorder such as PUD (Drossman et al., 1998; Engel, 1977). This model suggests that illness, "the subjective experience of feeling unwell," and disease, "an objective biological event of either tissue damage or associated organ malfunction," result from simultaneously interacting systems at the cellular, tissue, organismal, interpersonal, and environmental levels (Drossman, 1998; Engel, 1977). The biopsychosocial model is transactional, acknowledging the reciprocal influences of both biological and psychosocial factors. and it recognizes that the boundaries between health and disease are impacted by cultural, social, and psychological considerations (Gatchel, 2004; Lamberg, 2003). This model recognizes that "feeling well" is not the same thing as being healthy; for example, a serious disease such as hypertension can be fatal with few or no symptoms. Conversely, people cannot be healthy if they do not "feel well": if someone feels pain from a misperceived normal bodily sensation, the pain still hurts regardless of the source.

Data that document the comorbidity of mental and physical health problems, especially in chronic illnesses, reinforce that physical and psychological symptoms increase together: studies have demonstrated a correlation of 0.5 between psychological distress scales and physical symptoms (Watson & Pennebaker, 1989).

THE MIND/BODY RELATIONSHIP: A HISTORY OF GASTROINTESTINAL DISORDERS

Literature documents a long history identifying the relationship between emotional factors and gastrointestinal disorders; examples from Shakespeare to the present are replete with allusions to the GI tract being affected by an array of emotions. Contemporary language confirms this association with descriptive comments such as: "gut instinct," "became choked up," "nervous stomach," and "swallowed abuse."

Early information describing the relationship between gastrointestinal functioning and emotions began with the study of individuals who had sustained a gastrostomy, the surgical construction of a permanent opening from the external surface of the abdominal wall into the stomach. Beaumont (1959), in 1833, treated a man with a permanent gastric fistula sustained by a gunshot wound. He obtained objective data from the changes in the gastric fistula, linking emotionally charged experiences to the behavior of the stomach.

Beaumont's work stimulated further studies; Pavlov conducted perhaps the most famous of these studies, demonstrating in dogs the evoked secretory response, which occurred in anticipation of feeding. In the 1940s, Wolff conducted a case study of a man with a gastrostomy due to the burning of his esophagus at 9 years of age. Data from observations over a period of 20 years documented that his reactions to fright, depression, and being overwhelmed were associated with consistent and observable physiological changes in his stomach (Wolf, 1981). Since these earlier studies, more sophisticated neuroimaging techniques have been used to confirm the gut's responses to emotional factors (Derbyshire, 2003; Hobson & Aziz, 2004).

BIOPSYCHOSOCIAL MODEL AND PEDIATRIC GASTROINTESTINAL DISORDERS

Reports of gastrointestinal distress by children such as "my tummy hurts," "I feel like I'm going to throw up," or "I'm afraid it will hurt when I poop" are common childhood complaints voiced to parents and pediatricians. When traditional treatment methods used to manage these symptoms are not successful, the child and family are often referred to a pediatric gastroenterologist.

The problems and disorders seen in a pediatric GI practice are clinically challenging and range from the primarily functional in nature, such as recurrent abdominal pain (RAP), to those reflecting organic disease, such as Crohn's disease or ulcerative colitis. This broad range of pediatric GI problems is increasingly conceptualized from a biopsychosocial perspective. Interactions between physiological (e.g., motility, sensation) and psychological factors (e.g., life stress, emotional state, coping, social support) are seen as shaping the nature and outcome of the child's gastrointestinal symptoms. Factors such as the child's adoption of a sick role, their sensitivity to pain, their level of psychological functioning, and the family's ability to deal with the illness can all contribute to differences among children's reaction to illness (Drossman, 1998; Hyams, 1996).

Thus, for example, some adolescents with severe Crohn's disease do not limit their functioning and will not let the illness define them, participating in a wide range of academic and extracurricular activities. However, others with less severe physical symptoms but who are anxious and whose parents have significant concerns about their health status are home schooled and have little peer contact. A child with abdominal pain but with no psychosocial problems as well as good coping skills and social support will have a better outcome than the child with abdominal pain as well as coexisting emotional difficulties, high life stress, or limited support. Furthermore, the child's clinical outcome (e.g., daily function, quality of life) will, in turn, affect the severity of symptoms. This perspective stands in contrast to the conventional medical model, which is reductionist in nature and assumes that a patient with a symptom has a disease.

The biopsychosocial model elucidates two important issues with respect to pediatric GI disorders. The first is that illness factors related to pediatric GI disorders are not the sole cause of a child or adolescent's decline in functioning: psychological and environmental factors also have an important impact on functioning. The second is that helping the child and family cope with their responses to illness-related factors (e.g., painful symptoms, diagnostic testing, and complicated treatment regimens) is important so that age-appropriate development and functioning is not impaired. Early attention to possible psychosocial contributors increases opportunities to prevent maladaptive coping, adjustment difficulties, and associated disability.

The increase in health-related quality of life (HRQOL) studies in pediatric GI disorders, (Akobeng et al., 1999; Loonen, Grootenhuis, Last, & Derkx, 2004; Pace et al., 2003; Voskuijl et al., 2004; Cunningham, Drotar, Palermo McGowan, & Arendt, 2006), which assess a patient's outcome from a broader perspective than just disease measures, indicates the increasing recognition that "successful management of pediatric GI conditions should include measures of whether we improve our patient's quality of life" (Youssef, 2004, p. 461).

FUNCTIONAL GASTROINTESTINAL DISORDERS

Determining the relationship between physical and psychosocial factors is more complicated when physical symptoms such as cramping, abdominal pain, and fear of choking are present but physical findings from diagnostic tests are normal. Functional gastrointestinal disorders (FGIDs) are pediatric GI disorders in which variable combinations of chronic or recurrent GI symptoms (abdominal pain, bloating, the fear of choking, problems in the passage of food or feces, or any combination of these symptoms) predominate, but evidence of physical damage or abnormalities in the GI tract are not present (Hyams, 1999). FGIDs are linked by dysfunction of motility and in some disorders, sensory dysfunction of the gut. They exhibit shared features, including sensitivity to intestinal sensation, motility, and stress responses. From a biopsychosocial perspective, FGID symptoms represent the end product of the synthesis of a number of pathways: autonomic nervous system (ANS) reactivity and recovery, environmental stresses, the child's coping mechanisms, and parental responses to the child's symptoms.

FGIDs are prevalent and they are associated with significant work and school absenteeism, impaired HRQOL, and increased medical costs (Drossman et al., 1999; Lackner, Mesmer, Morley, Dowzer, & Hamilton, 2004; Walker, 1999). Routine activities of daily living may be curtailed for children and their families; in fact, disabilities due to FGIDs in children and for their families can equal or surpass organic GI problems, due to the uncertainty of the cause of the physical symptoms (Hyams, 1999).

Attempts to improve diagnosis and treatment of these complicated disorders have led to different conceptualizations of FGIDs. One schema is organized by focusing on issues of gastrointestinal motility, defined as the movements of the digestive system and the transit of the contents within it. Motility problems develop when nerves or muscles in any portion of the digestive tract do not function in a coordinated manner. Symptoms may range from heartburn to constipation and may also include abdominal distension, nausea, vomiting, and diarrhea (Locke, 1996).

Locke (1996) suggests that the distinctions between GI motility disorders and FGIDs are arbitrary. He proposes that motility disorders and FGIDs are not distinct diagnoses, but rather fall along a continuum, based upon the degree to which abnormal motility is thought to be involved in the pathogenesis of the disorder (Figure 2.1).

The most widely agreed-upon classification schema for pediatric FGIDs was developed in 1999 by experts in pediatric gastroenterology who met in Rome 7 years after FGIDs in adults were classified. The decision-making process for classification of pediatric FGIDs was the same as for adults: consensus for each FGID was based on clinical experience. However the classification system for children is organized by symptoms or complaints, reported by children or their parents/caregivers, whereas in adults, it is organized around targeted organs. This classification schema shifted the diagnostic process of FGIDs from an exclusionary diagnosis: the absence of organic problems, to one based upon the positive findings of specific symptoms. Consequently, the categorization of criteria for pediatric FGID's has provided

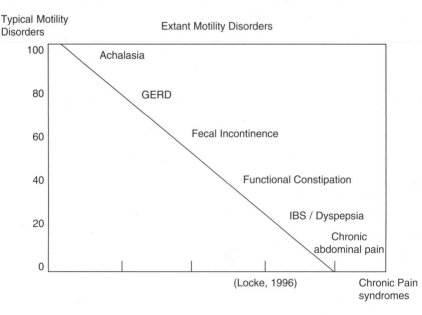

FIGURE 2.1. Extant Motility Disorders

TABLE 2.1. Classification of Functional Pediatric Gastrointestinal Disorders

1. Vomiting
   a. Infant regurgitation
   b. Infant rumination syndrome
   c. Cyclic vomiting syndrome

2. Abdominal pain
   a. Functional dyspepsia
   b. Irritable bowel syndrome
   c. Functional abdominal pain
   d. Abdominal migraine
   e. Aerophagia

3. Functional diarrhea

4. Disorders of defecation
   a. Infant dyschezia
   b. Functional constipation
   c. Functional fecal retention
   d. Nonretentive fecal soiling

Source: Rasquin-Weber et al., 1999.

a method of standardizing FGIDs, facilitating the study of these disorders from a variety of disciplines (Table 2.1).

In children FGIDs include combinations of often age-dependent, chronic, or recurrent symptoms not explained by structural or biochemical abnormalities (Rasquin-Weber et al., 1999) Some disorders may accompany normal development such as infant regurgitation, while others may represent a maladaptive response either to internal or external stimuli, for example, fecal retention due either to a painful bowel movement (internal stimuli) or to lack of comfort using the toilet at school (external stimuli). For certain disorders including irritable bowel syndrome (IBS) and functional dyspepsia, the criteria utilized in the adult population were replicated exactly for the pediatric population because they applied equally well for children. Pediatric FGIDs that utilize the adult criteria include: globus, functional chest pain, functional heartburn, functional dysphagia, and proctalgia fugax (Rasquin-Weber et al., 1999). The Rome group recognized that the co-occurrence of a FGID and organic disease in the same child could go unrecognized. Thus a child with inflammatory bowel disease (IBD) may be overtreated because of copresenting with IBS.

The Rome group postulated that a temperament characterized in part by gastrointestinal reactivity to stress is inherited by some infants and constitutes a genetic susceptibility to FGIDs. Twin studies support an underlying genetic predisposition in those with IBS. Concordance for functional bowel disorders was 33% for monozygotic twins versus 13% for dyzygotic twins (Levy et al., 2001). Two environmental factors are also reported to play a significant role in the development of FGID in children. The first is the plasticity of the neonatal brain, which may program early physiologic responses to stress during infancy and then continue into adulthood. The second factor includes illness-related behaviors and attitudes about "being sick" that children learn from their parents or caregivers (Whitehead, 1994). Studies document that health care utilization by children closely resembles that of their parents (Schor, Starfield, Stidley, & Hankin, 1987). Levy, Whitehead, Von Korff, and Feld (2000) evaluated early learning and heritability in the clinical expression of FGIDs in childhood. They reported a relationship between a parent's response to their child's illness and a child's disability from that illness. In a more recent study, Levy (2004) found that children with higher absentee levels for GI symptoms as reported by their mothers were more likely to have parents with IBS who were more solicitous to their child's symptoms. Our clinical experience corroborates these findings. Children's symptoms can become reinforced and persist even longer when parents focus on and pay too much attention to their children's pain and illness behavior. Children with RAP, whose parents are anxious themselves and who often visit physicians, are likely to have a greater number of diagnostic procedures, inpatient hospitalizations, and outpatient doctor visits. Additionally, interference with age-appropriate functioning due to pain complaints is more likely to be tolerated. For example, if the child reports that they are "too sick to go to school," parents, with a history of anxiety, are more likely let them stay home or they will pick the child up from school if the nurse calls.

The Rome II Criteria have been instrumental in defining diagnostic categories of Pediatric FGIDs and the specific criteria of these disorders. This schema has been an important step in the development of the consensual and systematic approach to these disorders in children and adolescents. However, recently studies have indicated that the Rome II criteria may be too restrictive pertaining to the prevalence of functional disorders related to constipation (Voskuijl, Heijmans, Heijmans, Taminiau, & Benninga, 2004). Efforts to validate the Pediatric Rome II criteria resulted in the development of the Questionnaire on Pediatric Gastrointestinal Symptoms (QPGS), a self-report questionnaire measuring the child's gastrointestinal symptoms (Caplan, Walker, & Rasquin, 2005). Its purpose is twofold: first, to aid pediatricians in diagnosing pediatric FGIDs and second, to serve as a research tool to estimate the incidence and the characteristics of these disorders. Further validation studies will contribute to the refinement of these diagnostic criteria and the systematic approach to these disorders in children.

It is worth noting that despite the fact that FGIDs account for the majority of visits to primary care physicians, functional gastrointestinal disorder research remains severely underfunded. Less than 1% of digestive disease research funding through the National Institutes of Health (NIH) is allocated for functional disorders (Gershon, 1998). Pace et al. (2003) cite a bias against irritable bowel syndrome (IBS), a functional disorder, considered by some physicians to be "all in the head" as compared to IBD, "a real disease," which is reflected in research funding. Despite the higher prevalence of IBS (10% of pediatric population for IBS versus pediatric data of 4.56/100,000 for Crohn's disease (CD), 2.24/100,000 for ulcerative colitis (UC), much greater resources are allocated to find a cure for IBD (Hyams, 1996; Kugathasan et al., 2003).

BRAIN-GUT INTERACTION

Studies examining FGIDs in children and adults have documented that stress and emotion impact physical symptoms in the gastrointestinal tract, from the esophagus to the rectum, and that there are intricate links between the nervous system and the digestive system (King, 2003; Pace et al., 2003; Walker, 1999; Whitehead, 1992). However, determining the pathways and the mechanisms of transmission of physical reactions to emotional situations and the reverse, emotional distress due to physical symptoms remains complicated. The conceptualization of FGIDs resulting from a brain-gut dysregulation is a hypothesis, which unifies the former dualistic concepts of mind/body issues (Wilhelmsen, 2000).

Recent progress toward a better understanding of these pathways and the transmission of information is due to two factors. First, research in the field of neurogastroenterology (the examination of the connections between the enteric nervous system and the central nervous system) has begun to delineate how these complicated pathways work and to increase our understanding of the impact of the mind/body relationship in the gastrointestinal tract. Second, there is an increase in scientific information regarding the gut's independent nervous system, the enteric nervous system (ENS).

History of Brain–Gut Interaction

The field of neurogastroenterology began with the work of Bayliss and Starling in England in the 1800s (Gershon, 1998). They isolated the intestine of a dog, stimulating the bowel from inside the intestine. Their experiments documented that digestion occurred even when the nerves to other organs in the body had been severed: the gut displayed reflex activity independent from the input of the central nervous system (CNS) (the brain and the spinal cord). They called the propulsive movement of the bowel in response to increased pressure, resulting in a coordinated wave of oral contractions and anal relaxation, the law of the intestine. In 1917, Trendelenburg (Gershon, 1998) observed the same phenomena in a loop of intestine that had been isolated from a guinea pig in an organ bath. He replaced the term law of the intestine with the term peristaltic reflex: the process by which motility in the gut proceeds without direction from the brain, spinal cord, or brainstem to the anus. Langley (Gershon, 1998), in the 1920s, described the autonomic nervous system (ANS) as a motor system of nerves that control the behavior of the visceral muscles, blood vessels, heart, and glands. He identified a third division in the ANS addition to the sympathetic and the parasympathetic, the ENS (Gershon, 1998).

The Enteric Nervous System

The ENS differs from the other two divisions in the ANS in its independence from the brain and the spinal cord. Typically commands flow from the brain via the nerves of the peripheral nervous system to muscles and glands (the effectors that do what the brain and spinal cord tell them to do). The enteric nervous system, however, does not respond in this hierarchical function. It is an independent site of neural integration and processing, which commands the gut by processing data by itself and then acts on the basis of this data. Once food is in the stomach, digestion and absorption can take place. The CNS is needed for swallowing and defecation—*in between the gut is in charge.*

The brain and the gut originate early in embryogenesis from the same clump of tissue, which divides during fetal development. The two nervous systems, the CNS and the ENS, are connected by the longest of the cranial nerves, the vagus nerve. This large "electrical cable" extends from the brainstem through the neck to the abdomen. The enteric nervous system is located in the sheaths of tissue that surround the linings of the organs of the GI tract: the esophagus, the stomach, the small intestine, and the colon. It is composed of two networks of neural connections: the mesenteric plexus and the submucosal plexus. These two networks are closely interconnected and they have their own complex circuitry, which provides the GI tract with the means to act independently. These network circuits are responsible for providing continuous back and forth interactions of information and feedback between the gut and the brain, thereby influencing brain and gut processes and gut functions (Blakeslee, 1996).

How the Brain–Gut Axis Works

The term brain-gut axis is used to explain the bidirectional neural pathways between the cognitive and emotional centers in the brain and the enteric nervous system in the gut (Buldavari & Olden, 2003). This bidirectional communication of a constant stream of chemical and electrical messages between the CNS and the ENS is increasingly acknowledged as the underlying pathomechanism of FGIDs (Gershon, 1998.) Chronic GI symptoms are a result of the integration of intestinal, motor, sensory, autonomic, and CNS activity, which interact at all levels of the brain-gut axis (Figure 2.2).

How does this process work? Because of the neural connections from the brain, circuits can be activated by external stimuli (a frightening event, stress, reactions to smell) or internal stimuli (bad thoughts or emotions), which can then alter motility and sensation in the gut. Because of the bidirectional nature of the brain-gut axis, the effect can work in reverse: the ENS sends signals to the brain as to what is occurring in the gut. Thus, physiological disturbances in the gut can affect mood, pain perception, and behavior.

How does the transmission of information actually occur? Communication between nerve cells is the basis of functioning for any part of the vertebrate system. The components of this processing system include neurotransmitters, hormones, and cytokines that act as messenger molecules carrying information between the nervous endocrine and immune systems. Information is passed from one site to another at the synapse level with the aid of neurotransmitters. The flow of information going from the brain to the gut and the gut to the brain is regulated by a variety of neurotransmitters

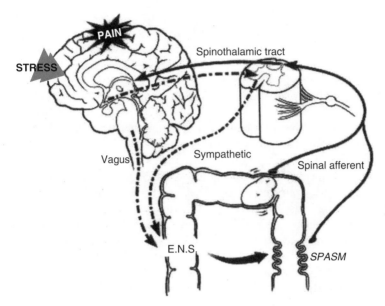

FIGURE 2.2. Brain–gut axis mechanism (Mertz, 2003)

found in both the brain and the gut. Serotonin, a brain neurotransmitter and a mediator of the brain-gut connection, is used as an antidepressant in a class of drugs called SSRIs (selective serotonin reuptake inhibitors). These drugs are thought to ease depression by increasing the amount of serotonin in the brain, yet 95% of the body's serotonin is stored and manufactured in the bowel (Kim & Camilleri, 2000). Does this class of drugs actually work on the gut, not the brain, to improve mood?

New diagnostic procedures have aided in the confirmation of this brain-gut link. Neuroimaging procedures such as computed tomography (CT) scan, positron emission tomography (PET), and functional magnetic resonance imaging (fMRI) are noninvasive imaging techniques used to examine how specific areas of the brain perform in response to visceral sensation (Derbyshire, 2003). This technology has clarified the relationship between specific regions of the brain and the functions they perform in response to stimuli.

The Brain–Gut Interaction and Irritable Bowel Syndrome

Recent research by Hamaguchi et al. (2004) supports a brain-gut relationship as a major factor in the pathophysiology of IBS. They reported findings of distension of the descending colon, which induces visceral perception and emotion, and correlates significantly with activation of specific regions of the brain including the limbic system and the association cortex, especially the prefrontal cortex. Their findings indicate that the brain has a specific functional module for response to visceral perception and perception-related emotion. Budavari and Olden (2003) suggest that variable influences of stress on gut function as mediated through neurotransmitter release may explain varied presentations of IBS. Studies using fMRI show that people with IBS process pain differently from controls: painful rectal distension prompts greater activation of their anterior cingulate cortex, a critical pain center.

Children and adolescents with IBS have visceral hypersensitivity, a heightened sensitivity of the nerves that go from the colon to the spinal cord. They may perceive colonic sensations differently from those children without IBS. For example, they may complain of incomplete evacuation even though their rectum is empty, or they may feel distended with gas even though when measured there is no significant increase in gas. Children with IBS may have fears in the morning about exams or social issues, which can precipitate cramping or just abnormal visceral sensitivity to normal bodily functions. Their cramping causes anxiety about having to go to school: What if they have excess flatulence? What if they have to use the toilet? These concerns can lead to school avoidance, which then increases the child's feelings of pressure because of being behind in classes. Mach (2004) reported that to date scientific evidence supporting traditional therapies have been limited and that understanding the brain–gut axis is crucial in the development of new effective therapies in the management for IBS.

Figure 2.3 is a visual representation of a biopsychosocial approach to IBS, which encompasses the transactional relationship between the CNS and the ENS. This model integrates factors that lead to IBS and the transactional

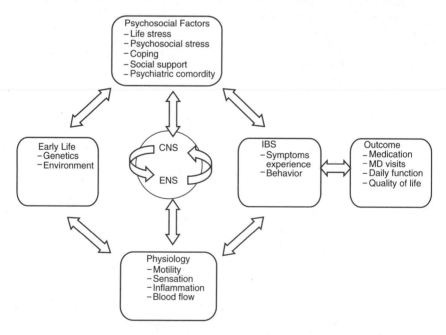

FIGURE 2.3. Biopsychosocial model of IBS depicting the relationship between early life, psychological factors, physiology, subjective experience ENS-enteric nervous system (Mulak & Bonaz, 2004)

process by which these factors affect each other, resulting in the expression of IBS in the child or adolescent. Early life factors (e.g., genetic predisposition to GI disorders) interact with physiological factors (e.g., increased visceral sensitivity in the colon, diarrhea, and cramping) and psychosocial factors (e.g., stresses such as academic and social pressures, family conflicts, comorbid anxiety) to contribute to the diagnosis of IBS. A significant feature of this schema is the outcome: How do the child and the families react once a diagnosis of IBS is made? Is IBS the focus of the child's and the family's home life? Are daily age-appropriate activities such as school, athletics, and sleepovers limited because of fears of cramping, possible incontinence, or worries about vomiting? Does the child then limit his or her functioning in response to these physical concerns? Does the child sense the parent's anxiety and then become anxious? The transactional aspect of this process is critical and unique to each child or adolescent.

This bidirectional neural pathway between the CNS and the ENS affects children and adolescents with the whole spectrum of GI disorders. King (2003) reported that the reciprocal brain-gut relationship is also seen in children and adolescents with IBD. He reported that in one direction, stress can affect physical symptoms and in the other direction, he stated that having IBD and thoughts associated with the treatment and the symptoms can impact mood.

The brain–gut theory has sparked interest as well as controversy regarding the relationship between GI symptoms and autism, a life long disorder characterized by problems with communication, socialization, and abnormal responses to sensations, including pain. For a long time, GI symptoms in children with autism had been overlooked or attributed to the behaviors (aching, flailing, and biting) and sensory dysfunction associated with autism. While parental reports, case studies, and small uncontrolled trials have reported a relationship between GI issues in children and autism, research has documented mixed results. (Erickson et al., 2005).

Several population studies have examined the prevalence of GI symptoms in children with autism. Studies report that 46–76% of children with autism have overt GI symptoms compared to 10–30% of typically developing developmentally pediatric controls (Horvath & Perman, 2002; Wakefield, 2002). The most commonly reported symptoms include chronic diarrhea, constipation, abdominal bloating, food sensitivities, and food regurgitation (Wakefield, 2002; Molloy et al., 2003). Horvath (1999) and Kushak (2002) also have documented an increase in the incidence of lactose and sugar intolerances in children with autism as compared to controls.

The history linking autism and GI disorders began with the original description of autism by Kanner (1943), who reported that 6 of the 11 children identified with this disorder had feeding difficulties. In the 1950s and 1960s, researchers evaluated diet and food allergies as a trigger for autism. Studies by Prugh (1951), Daynes (1951), and Asperger (1961) identified abnormal behaviors in children with gluten sensitivity or celiac sprue. Early studies by Crook (1961) reported cases of profound neurological behaviors including autism, which resolved with dietary changes, suggesting food allergies as a contributory factor. Goodwin (1971) described improvements in the EEG studies of randomly selected children with autism when the children were placed on gluten-free diets. These earlier studies, however, were based on case reports and anecdotal descriptions.

Several hypotheses have been proposed to explain the linkage between the GI tract and the brain in children with autism. These include the opioid theory, irregular secretin levels, and autoimmune dysfunction. The opioid theory asserts that autism is the result of a metabolic disorder (Shattock, 1990; Reichelt, 1991), in which peptides derived from dietary sources, in particular foods that contain gluten and casein, are mixed with digestive enzymes, resulting in opioid peptides. These peptides pass through an abnormally permeable intestinal membrane ("leaky gut") and enter the CNS, causing neurological dysfunction or encephalopathic issues. Yet, in contrast to the large amount of parental anecdotal information and case studies, Erickson et al. (2005) in a review report that "overall studies analyzing the response of autistic children to dietary proteins have found mixed results" (p. 21).

Secretin has also been reported as a possible link to the GI-autism issue. Horvath et al. (1998) documented the improvement in three children with autism with respect to their GI issues as well as their eye contact, alertness, and expressive language after receiving IV secretin during a GI procedure. They hypothesized that the low level of secretin, which has an effect on gastric secretion, contributed to an increased incidence of acid reflux and perhaps pain-related behaviors. However, further studies that examined providing IV secretion to children with autism have not resulted in improvement in GI symptoms or autistic behaviors (White, 2003).

Recently studies have examined the histopathology of the GI tract in children with autism. These studies support the presence of chronic inflammation in the GI tract with the possibility of an autoimmune process contributing to the inflammatory response. Wakefield et al. (2000) undertook a systematic evaluation of GI symptoms in children with autism. Colonoscopy revealed that 93% of the children had ileo lymphoid nodular hyperplasia. Furante (2001), Torrente (2002), and Ashwood (2004) have reported immune abnormalities and abnormal cytokine profiles, inflammatory markers in children with autism who have GI symptoms. Jyonouchi, Greg, Ruby, Reddy, and Zimmerman-Bier (2005) documented a defect of innate immune responses in children with autism with GI symptoms but not in children with nonallergic food hypersensitivity or children with autism without GI symptoms, suggesting a possible link between GI and behavioral symptoms mediated by innate immune abnormalities. This subgroup of children with autism and GI symptoms may not be able to resist exposure to benign dietary, triggers, which may increase behavioral symptoms.

Attempts to further understand the connections between children with autism who have GI symptoms have led to identifying different subgroups among this population. D'Eufemia et al. (1996) reported that 43% of children with autism tested had increased gut permeability but no history of GI symptoms. Molloy and Manning-Courtney (2003) found that in a study of a general population of children with autism, 24% had a history of one chronic GI symptom, most commonly diarrhea (21%). Molloy and Manning-Courtney (2003) speculated that these children might represent a distinct phenotypic subgroup within the larger group of children who meet the criteria for autism. In light of D'Eufemia's findings, they propose a continuum of children with autism and presenting GI symptoms to include normal/ asymptomatic to abnormal/asymptomatic to abnormal/symptomatic as a paradigm for differentiating among subtypes of children with autism who have GI issues.

To date, research and parental report document that GI symptoms in certain subgroups of children with autism exist; however, a causative relationship has not been empirically documented. Behaviors associated with autism may have a variety of origins: attention seeking, self stimulation, frustration with inability to communicate, and pain that may have medical underpinnings. GI issues may exacerbate autistic symptoms; thus the treatment of GI issues may not only heal the GI symptoms but may also decrease problem behaviors in children with autism. As research continues to clarify the brain–gut connection in children with autism, GI symptoms in this population need to be carefully evaluated and treated.

In the process of examining a theoretical basis for pediatric GI disorders we have come full circle: from the Greek theory of holos (integration of psyche and soma) to dualist conceptualizations of illness, and finally to examining the brain-gut axis as a unifying principle. We end this chapter with a prescient quote from an 18th-century physician and chemist:

> Finally the mind itself and the body, things generally held to be of entirely disparate nature, are so tightly and intimately knit when joined together in man that—if I may here speak as a chemist—they interpenetrate and dissolve in each other, so that while life flourishes, wherever there is mind there is body, and wherever body, mind. There is hardly to be found any smallest part of man in which something of the mind and something of the body, and in measure a mixture of both, is not to be observed. (Jacob Gaub, in Rather, p. 34, 1965).

Simply put, the brain affects the gut and the gut can affect the brain.

The following chapters focus on the assessment and treatment of the following pediatric gastrointestinal disorders: inflammatory bowel disease (IBD), recurrent abdominal pain (RAP), vomiting disorders, esophageal disorders (globus sensation, gastroesophagal reflux (GER), gastroesophageal reflux disease (GERD), irritable bowel syndrome (IBS), and defecation disorders. For each of the disorders discussed, we will present:

1. Our clinical experience in terms of assessing and treating these disorders.
2. What we know from evidenced-based research about the treatment of these disorders. What data report regarding which psychosocial treatments work best with which pediatric GI disorder.
3. The roadblocks in treating these pediatric GI disorders from a biopsychosocial perspective.

Our goal is to clarify what is known with respect to the psychological and behavioral assessment and treatment of pediatric GI disorders and to elucidate the areas in need of further investigation.

REFERENCES

Akobeng, A. K., Suresh-Babu, M. V., Firth, D., Miller, V., Mir, P., & Thomas, A. G. (1999). Quality of life in children with Crohn's disease: A pilot study. *Journal of Pediatric Gastroenterology Nutrition, 4*, 37–39.

Ashwood, P., Anthony, A., Pellier, A. A., Torrente, F., Walker-Smith, J. A., & (2003). Wakefield A. J.: Intestinal lymphocyte population in children with regressive autism: Evidence for extensive muscosal immunopathology, *Journal Clinical Immunology, 23*, 504–517.

Beaumont, W. (1959). *Experiments and observation on the gastric juice and the physiology of digestion.* New York: Dover. (Originally published in 1833)

Blakeslee, S. (1996, January 23). Complex hidden brain in gut makes bellyaches and butterflies. *New York Times*, p. c1.

Budavari, A. I., & Olden, K. W. (2003, June). Psychosocial aspects of functional gastrointestinal disorders. *Gastoenterology Clinics of North America, 32*(2), 477–506.

Caplan, A., Walker, L., Rasquin, A. (2005). Development and preliminary validation of the questionnaire of pediatric gastrointestinal syndroms to assess functional gastrointestinal in children and adolescents. *Journal Pediatric Gastroenterology and Nutrition, 41*(3), 296–304.

Cunningham, C., Drotar, D., Palermo, T., McGowan, K., Arendt, R. (2006). Health related quality of life in children and adolescents with inflammatory bowel disease. *Submitted manuscript.*

Defelice, M. L., Ruchelli, E. D., Markowitz, J. E., Strogatz, M., Reddy, K. P., & Kadivar, K. et al. (2003). Intestinal cytokines in children with pervasive developmental disorders. *American Journal of Gastroenterology, 98*, 1777–1782.

D'Eufemia, P., Celli, M., Fincchiaro, R., Pacifico, L., Viozzi, L., & Zaccagnini, M. et al. (1996). Abnormal intestinal permeability in children with autism. *Acta Paediatrics, 85*, 1076–1079.

Derbyshire, S. W. (2003). A systematic review of neuroimaging data during visceral stimulation. *American Journal of Gastroenterology, 98*(1), 12–20.

Drossman, D. A. (1998). Presidential address: Gastrointestinal illness and the biopsychosocial model. *Pyschosomatic Medicine, 60*(3), 258–267.

Drossman, D., Creed, F. H., Olden, K. W., Svedlund, J., Toner, B. B., & Whitehead, W. E. (1999). Psychosocial aspects of the functional gastrointestinal disorders. *Gut, 45*(Suppl. II), II25–II30.

Dunbar, F. (1954). *Emotions and bodily changes.* New York: Columbia University Press.

Engel, G. L. (1977). The need for a new medical model: A challenge for biomedicine. *Science, 196*, 129–136.

Entralgo, P. L. (1956). *Mind and body.* New York: Kennedy and Sons.

Erickson, C. A., Stigler, K. A., Corkins, M. R., Posey, D., Fitzgerald, J. F., & McDougle, C. J. (2005). Gastrointestinal factors in autistic disorder: A critical review. *Journal of Autism and Developmental Disorders, 4*, 1–15.

Finney, J. W., Lemanek, K. L., Cataldo, M. F., Katz, H. P., & Fuqua, R. W. (1989). Pediatric psychology in primary health care: Brief targeted therapy for recurrent abdominal pain. *Behavior Therapy, 20*, 283–291.

Gatchel, R. J. (2004). Comorbidity of chronic pain and mental health disorders: The biopsychosocial perspective. *American Psychologist, 59*(8), 795–805.

Gershon, M. D. (1998). *The second brain.* New York: Harper Collins.

Hamaguchi, T., Kano, M., Rikimaru, H., Kanazawa, M., Itoh, M., Yanai, K. et al. *Neurogastroenterology and Motility, 16*(3), 299–309.

Hobson, A. R., & Aziz, Q. (2004, August). Brain imaging and functional gastrointestinal disorders: Has it helped our understanding? *Gut, 53*(8), 1198–1206.

Horvath, K., Papadimitriou, J. C., Rabsztyn, A., Drachenberg, C., & Tildon, J. T. (1999). Gastrointestinal abnormalities in children with autistic disorder. *Journal of Pediatrics, 135*, 559–563.

Horvath, K., & Perman, J. A. (2002). Autistic disorder and gastrointestinal disease. *Current Opinion in Pediatrics, 14,* 583–587.

Horvath, K., Stefanatos, G., Sokolski, K. N., Luachtel, R., Nabors, L., Tildon, J. T. et al. (1998). Improved social and language skills after secretion administration in patients with autistic spectrum disorders. *Journal of Association of Academic Minority Physicians, 9*, 9–15.

Hyams, J. S. (1996). Crohn's disease in children. *Pediatric Clinics of North America, 43*, 255–277.

Hyams, J. S. (1999). Functional gastrointestinal disorders. *Current Opinions in Pediatrics, 11*(5), 375–378.

Hyams, J. S. (2002). *Pediatric functional gastrointestinal disorders.* New York: Academy Professional Information Services.

Jyonouchi, H., Greg, L., Ruby, A., Reddy, C., & Zimmerman-Bier, B. (2005). Evaluation of an association between gastrointestinal symptoms and cytokine production against common dietary protiens in children with autism spectrum disorders. *Journal of Pediatrics, 146*, 605–610.

Jyonouchi, H., Sun, S., & Itokazu, N. (2002). Innate immunity associated with inflammatory responses and cytokine production against common dietary proteins in patients with autism spectrum disorder. *Neuropsychobiology, 46*, 76–84.

Kim, D. Y., & Camilleri, M. (2000). Serotonin: A mediator of the brain-gut connection. *American Journal of Gastroenterology, 95*(10), 2698–2709.

King, R. A. (2003, July). Pediatric inflammatory bowel disease. *Child and Adolescent Psychiatric Clinics of North America, 12*(3), 537–550.

Kugathasan, S., Judd, R. H., Hoffman, N. R. G. Heikenen, J., Telega, G. et al. (2003). Epidemologic and clinical characteristics of children with newly diagnosed inflammatory bowel disease in Wisconsin. *Journal of Pediatrics, 143*(4), 523–531.

Lackner, J. M., Mesmer, C., Morley, S., Dowzer, C., & Hamilton, S. (2004). Psychological treatments for irritable bowel syndrome: a systematic review and meta-analysis. *Journal of Consulting and Clinical Psychology, 72*(6), 1100–1113.

Lamberg, L. (2003, July 24–31). Mind-body medicine explored at APA meeting. *Journal of the American Medical Association, 288*(4), 335–337.

Levenstein, S. (2000). The very model of a modern etiology: A biopsychosocial view of peptic ulcer disease. *Psychosomatic Medicine, 62*, 176–185.

Levy, R. L., Whitehead, W. E., Von Korff, M., & Feld, A. D. (2000). Intergenerational transmission of gastrointestinal illness behavior. *American Journal of Gastroenterology, 95*(2), 451–456.

Levy, R., Jones, K., Whitehead, W., Feld, S., Talley, N., Corey, L. (2001). Irritable bowel syndrome in twins: Heredity and social learning both contribute to etiology. *Journal of American Gastroenterology Association Institute, 121*(4), 799–804.

Levy, R., Whitehead, W., Walker, S., Von Korff, M., Feld, A., Garner, M., Christie, D. (2004). Increased somatic complaints and health-care utilization in children: Effects of parent IBS status and parent response to gastrointestinal symptoms. *American Journal of Gastroenterology, 99*(12), 1–10.

Locke, R. G. (1996). Epidemiology of functional gastrointestinal disorders in North America. *Gastroenterology Clinics of North America, 25*(1), 1–19.

Loonen, H. J., Grootenhuis, M. A., Last, B. F., & Derkx, H. H. F. (2004). Coping strategies and quality of life of adolescents with inflammatory bowel disease. *Quality of Life Research, 13*, 1011–1019.

Mach, T. (2004). The brain-gut axis in irritable bowel syndrome–clinical aspects. *Medical Science Monitor, 10*(6), RA125–31.

Mertz, H. R. (2003). Overview of functional gastrointestinal disorders: Dysfunction of the brain-gut axis. *Gastroenterology Clinics of North America, 32*, 463–476.

Molloy, C. A., & Manning-Courtney, P. (2003). Prevalence of chronic gastrointestinal symptoms in children with autism and autistic spectrum disorders. *Autism, 7*(2), 165–71.

Mulak, A., & Bonaz, B. (2004). Irritable bowel syndrome: A model of the brain-gut interactions. *Medical Science Monitor, 10*(4), RA55–62.

Nemiah, J. C. (2000, May–June). A psychodynamic view of psychomatic medicine. *Psychosomatic Medicine, 62*(3), 299–303.

Pace, F., Molteni, P., Bollani, S., Sarzi-Puttini, P., Stockbrugger, R., Bianchi Porro, G. et al. (2003). Inflammatory bowel disease versus irritable bowel syndrome: A hospital based, case-control study of disease impact on quality of life. *Scandinavian Journal of Gastroenterology, 38*(10), 31–38.

Perkin, G. D., & Murray-Lyon, I. (1998, September). Review of *Neurology and the gastrointestinal system. Journal of Neurology, Neurosurgery, and Psychiatry, 65*(3), 291–300.

Rasquin-Weber, A., Hyman, P. E., Cucchiara, S., Fleisher, D. R., Hyams, J. S., Milla, P. J. et al. (1999). Childhood functional gastrointestinal disorders. *Gut, 45*(Suppl. II), II60–II68.

Rather L. J. (1965). *Mind and body in eighteenth-century medicine: A study based on Jerome Gaub De Regime-Mentis.* Berkeley: University of California Press.

Ray, O. (2004). How the mind hurts and heals the body. *American Psychologist, 59*(1), 29–40.

Rayhorn, N. (2001). Treatment of inflammatory bowel disease in the adolescent. *Journal of Infusion Nursing, 24*(4), 255–262.

Reichelt, K. L., Ekrein, J., & Scott, H. (1990). Gluten, milk proteins, and autism: Dietary intervention effects on behavior and peptide secretion. *Journal of Applied Nutrition, 42*, 1–11.

Ringdahl, I. C. (1980). Hospital treatment of the encopretic child. *Psychosomatics.* January, 1,65,69–71.

Roccatagliata, G. (1997). Classical psychopathology. In W. G. Bringman et al. (Eds.), *A pictorial history of psychology* (pp. 383–390). Chicago: Quintessence Publishing.

Schor, E., Starfield, B., Stidley, C., & Hankin, J. (1987). Family health: Utilization and effects of family membership. *Medical Care, 25*(7), 616–626.

Torrente, F., Ashwood, P., Day, R., Machado, N., Furlano, R., Anthony, A. et al. (2002). Small intestinal enteropathy with epithelial IgG and complement deposition in children with regressive autism. *Molecular Psychiatry, 7*, 375–382.

Turk, D. C., & Monarch, E. S. (2002). Biopsychosocial perspective on chronic pain. In D. C. Turk & R. J. Gatchel (Eds.), *Psychological approaches to pain management: A practioner's handbook* (2nd ed., pp. 3–32). New York: Guilford.

Voskuijl, W. P., van der Zaag-Loonen, H. J., Ketel, I. J. G., Grootenhuis, M. A., Derkx, B. H. B., & Benninga, M. A. (2004). Health related quality of life in disorders of defecation: The defecation disorder list. *Archives of Disease in Childhood, 89*, 1124–1127.

Voskuijl, W. P., Heijmans, J., Heijmans, H. S., Taminiau, J. A., Benninga, M. A. (2004). Use of Rome II criteria in childhood defecation disorders: Applicability in clinical and research practice. *Pediatrics, 145*(2), 213–217.

Wakefield, A. J. (2002). The gut–brain axis in childhood developmental disorders. *Journal of Pediatrics Gastroenterology and Nutrition, 34*, S14–S17.

Wakefield, A. J., Anthony, A., Murch, S. H., Thomson, M., Montgomery, S. M., Davies, S. et al. (2000). Enterocolitis in children with developmental disorders. *American Journal of Gastroenterology, 95*, 2285–2295.

Walker, L. S. (1999, October). Pathways between recurrent abdominal pain and adult functional gastrointestinal disorders. *Journal of Developmental and Behavioral Pediatrics, 20*(5), 320–322.

Watson, D., & Pennebaker, J. (1989). Health complaints, stress, and distress: Exploring the central role of negative affectivity. *Psychological Review, 96*, 234–254.

White, J. F. (2003). Intestinal pathophysiology in autism. *Experimental Biology and Medicine, 228*(6), 639–647.

Whitehead, W. E. (1992). Behavioral medicine approaches to gastrointestinal disorders. *Journal of Consulting and Clinical Psychology, 60*(4), 605–612.

Whitehead, W. E., Crowell, M. D., Heller, B. R., Robinson, J. C., Schuster, M. M., & Horn, S. (1994, November–December). Modeling and reinforcement of the sick role during childhood predicts adult illness behavior. *Psychsomatic Medicine, 56*(6), 541–550.

Wilhelmsen, I. (2000). Brain-gut axis as an example of the biopsychosocial model. *Gut, 47*(Suppl. IV), IV5–IV7.

Wolf, S. (1981). The psyche and the stomach. *Gastroenterology, 80*(3), 605–614.

Youssef, N. (2004). IBD or IBS: When there is abdominal pain, does it really matter? *Journal of Pediatric Gastroenterology and Nutrition, 38*, 460–461.

Inflammatory Bowel Disease | 3

Inflammatory bowel disease (IBD) is an inflammatory disease of the digestive tract, which includes three distinct diagnoses categories: ulcerative colitis (UC), Crohn's disease (CD) and indeterminate colitis (IC). IBD is characterized by symptoms of abdominal pain, fatigue, weight loss, diarrhea, cramping, and joint pain. These symptoms often interfere with everyday life and can have long-term effects, such as delayed sexual maturity and growth retardation. In CD, the inflammation extends through the full thickness of the intestinal wall, and this inflammation may affect any part of the GI tract from the mouth to the skin around the anus. In UC, the inflammation is confined to the large intestine, and it is restricted to the inner lining of the colon. Figures 3.1 and 3.2 diagram the different areas of inflammation in CD and UC in children.

It is not known whether UC and CD are two distinct diseases that have similar clinical manifestations or causally related diseases that have different histopathologic and geographic localizations (Hyams, 1996; King, 2003). Patients who have a definite histological diagnosis of colitis but without a clear distinction between CD and UC are diagnosed with IC until the evolution of the disease allows for better differentiation (Rice & Chuang, 1999).

Inflammatory bowel disease (IBD) and irritable bowel syndrome (IBS) are often confused because they share common symptoms: abdominal pain, cramping, a sense of urgency, and diarrhea. They are, however, two separate disorders with different etiologies, different treatment regimens, and different long-term effects (see Table 3.1).

IBS, which is a functional GI disorder (Rasquin-Weber et al., 1999), does not cause bowel inflammation and bears no relationship to Crohn's disease or ulcerative colitis. Many patients with IBD are initially misdiagnosed with IBS and consequently believe that their symptoms are due to psychological factors, not a physical illness. For the patient with IBD, the nonspecific symptoms of abdominal pain and diarrhea may easily be mistaken for IBS, thus delaying the diagnosis. This is particularly true for CD where growth failure, arthrealgias, or fevers may be the sole presenting complaint. Until more recently, this resulted in the delay of a diagnosis from the time of presentation of symptoms since many of the presenting symptoms of CD (anorexia, fatigue, and abdominal pain complaints) were thought to be evidence of psychological, not physical, problems. Patients diagnosed with CD often initially report relief, knowing that a physical illness was causing their symptoms, despite having to accept the reality of having a chronic illness.

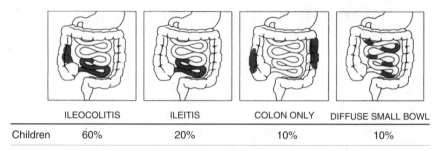

	ILEOCOLITIS	ILEITIS	COLON ONLY	DIFFUSE SMALL BOWL
Children	60%	20%	10%	10%

FIGURE 3.1. Distribution of Inflammation in Children with Crohn's Disease (Benkov & Winter, 1966)

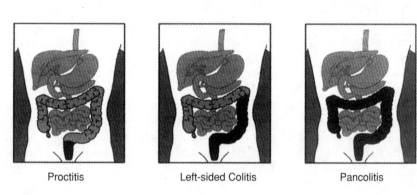

| Proctitis | Left-sided Colitis | Pancolitis |

FIGURE 3.2. Distribution of Inflammation in Children with ulcerative colitis (Benkov & Winter, 1966)

Children and adolescents diagnosed with IBD present with unique features, which require awareness of the diverse psychobiologic effects of the disorder over the course of their development. First, the disease symptoms and the treatment side effects can impact children's physical growth and maturation, consequently affecting their psychosocial development. Second, IBD raises considerations regarding the complex interactions between stress and the immune, endocrine, and the nervous systems. Third, pediatric IBD presents physicians and behavioral specialists with the challenge of providing comprehensive care in the time of declining resources for services (King, 2003).

EPIDEMIOLOGY

Population-based studies suggest that IBD is unevenly distributed throughout the world, with the highest disease rates occurring in first world, Westernized countries (Pappa, Semrin, Walker, & Grand, 2004) and the rates of IBD are

TABLE 3.1. Characteristics of IBD versus IBS in Children and Adolescents

	IBD	IBS

Symptoms	1. Abdominal pain/cramping
	2. Weight loss
	3. Fatigue
	4. Diarrhea
	5. Blood in stool
	6. Extraintestinal symptoms
	   a. Joint pain
	   b. Delayed growth
	   c. Anemia
		1. Abdominal pain or discomfort
		2. Changes in bowel habits
		3. Passage of mucous
		4. Bloating or feeling of abdominal distention

Prevalence	300,000 children and adolescents Crohn's disease: 4.56 per 100,000 Ulcerative colitis: 2.14 per 100,000 (Kugathasan et al., 2003) Indeterminate 15% of all pediatric colitis: IBD patients (King, 2003)	6–14% of adolescents (Hyams, Burke, Davis, Rzepsaki, & Andrulonis, 1996)

Etiology	1 Multifactorial including:
	   a. Genetic factors
	   b. Infectious factors
	   c. Immunological factors
	   d. No data supporting psychological, dietary etiology (Mamula et al., 2003)
		1. No structural or metabolic abnormalities to explain the symptoms
		2. Psychosocial factors (e.g., life stress, psychological state, coping, social support) interact with physiologic factors (e.g., motility, sensation) in the etiology of symptoms (Drossman, 2000)

Treatment		
Medical	1. Medication 2. Nutritional therapy 3. Surgery	1. Medication 2. Nutritional therapy
Psychological	1. Education 2. Proactive psychological intervention at strategic points in illness course 3. Support groups	1. Relaxation Training/biofeedback 2. Cognitive-behavioral stress management 3. Pain/behavior management 4. Training for parents

rising with urbanization (Hyams, 1996). The incidence of IBD is bimodal: the first peak occurs in the first to second decades of life, with the second rise noted between the fifth to seventh decades (Mamula, Markowitz, & Baldassano, 2003). IBD is diagnosed during childhood or adolescence in 25% to 30% of patients (Cuffari & Darbari, 2002; Kugathasan et al., 2003). IBD has been increasing since 1960, particularly in the pediatric population (Gryboski, 1994; Korelitz, 1982).

A unique aspect of IBD in children is a recent threefold increase in new cases of CD, whereas the incidence of UC has remained stable. A statewide population-based study in Wisconsin examined the epidemiological and clinical characteristics of children with newly diagnosed IBD (Kugathasan et al., 2003). The results indicated the highest pediatric IBD incidence reported in the world to date, a twofold predominance in pediatric CD incidence compared with UC, a significantly higher rate of CD diagnosis among boys compared to girls, a low frequency of patients with positive family histories, no modulatory effect of urbanization on pediatric IBD incidence, and equal distribution of IBD incidence among all ethnic populations. Kugathsan et al. (2003) suggest that because pediatric IBD now afflicts all races and ethnicities as well as rural and urban populations with a similar frequency, data underscore changing environmental factors as increasingly important factors in the pathogenesis of IBD. A recent prospective population-based study in northern France assessed the incidence of CD and UC in children and adolescents between 1988–1999. The results indicated an increasing trend in the incidence of CD, while the incidence of UC remained stable (Auvin et al., 2005). There has also been an increase in the number of patients diagnosed with IC (Cuffari & Darbari, 2002). Patients with IC account for approximately 15% of the cases of IBD that present as colitis (King, 2003).

Males and females are equally affected with respect to UC—for those 10–19 years of age the incidence rate is 2.3 per 100,000; however, a slight increase in incidence of CD in boys has recently been reported (Mamula et al., 2003). It is rare for UC to be diagnosed before the age of 5 (Langholz, Munkholm, Krasilnikoff, Binder, 1997). The incidence of CD is 5 to 10 per 100,000 people per year. The peak frequency of new CD cases in the pediatric population occurs in the mid- to late teens, with an age-specific incidence rate of approximately 16 per 100,000 (Hyams, 1996).

Disease incidence is clearly higher in first-degree relatives of individuals afflicted with IBD, with increased disease probability correlating with the number of first-degree relatives affected. Heyman et al. (2005) have recently documented that positive family history was especially common in young patients with UC. Americans of Jewish ancestry are known to have a rate of incidence three times higher than the national average. Young children with IBD are thought to be a unique subset of pediatric patients with IBD: these children are often reported to be more symptomatic than older children and adults. However, a case review of pediatric patients diagnosed with IBD reported that except for higher platelet counts, a lower body mass index, and a higher frequency of positive family history in young children with CD, there were no significant differences in the presentation of young children with IBD compared with older children (Weinstein et al., 2003).

ETIOLOGY

The etiology of IBD is unknown. Current theories propose a multifactorial etiology; the pathogenesis of the illness proceeds from a genetic predisposition (susceptible host) being exposed to specific triggers (e.g., bacteria, viruses,

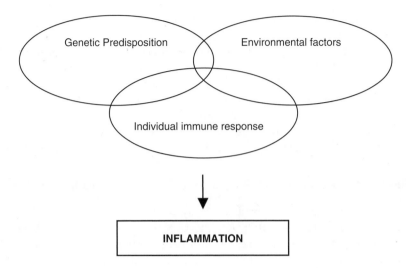

FIGURE 3.3. Interactive elements contributing to the pathogenesis of inflammatory bowel disease (Cunningham, 2002)

parasites, toxins, chemicals), which interact with the body's immune system and trigger the disease (see Figure 3.3.).

Advances in genetic testing have confirmed the presence of susceptibility loci on chromosomes 12 and 16 for UC and CD. These loci show a strong association with particular disease phenotypes that may explain the clinical heterogeneity of IBD (Cuffari & Darbari, 2002). A report based on a study of 90 pedigrees in the United States has demonstrated that linkage with IBD1 is greatest in pedigrees that include individuals who developed CD during childhood and who had more severe disease activity (Brandt et al., 2000). Linkage studies have also shown that a locus on chromosome 12 appears to affect UC susceptibility (Kim & Ferry, 2002). Although this genetic information may aid in the identification of patients with IBD, the lack of clear heritability reinforces the fact that the disease pathogenesis of IBD depends on the interaction between environmental factors and genetics. Baron et al. (2005) examined environmental risk factors prior to the development of IBD in a pediatric population case control study from a large registry in France. Their results indicated having a first-degree relative with IBD represents the single biggest risk factor in determining the disease. While recognizing the clear evidence for genetic susceptibility, Baron et al. questioned why there is geographic variation in disease incidence and why there is a rapid rise of CD over the past century. Their results led them to hypothesize that while family history and appendectomy are known risk factors, certain vaccinations, living arrangements, and dietary factors may lead to new etiological information.

Although data do not support a psychological etiology, such as stress or depression, the increasing incidence of CD has led to speculation about changes in exposure to environmental or infectious agents. Considerable attention has focused on the role of measles infection or vaccination in the pathogenesis of CD and UC. The World Health Organization conducted a thorough review of the literature and reported no direct correlation between measles virus or vaccines and IBD (Afzal et al., 1998). Finally, there is no definitive data to support diet as a cause of either CD or UC (Bremner & Beattie, 2002).

Relationship between Psychological Variables and IBD

Clinicians recognize the importance of psychosocial factors for pediatric and adolescent patients with IBD; yet, the hypothesized relationship between IBD and psychological variables has not been supported by evidence-based research. Prior studies reported that psychological conflict such as unexpressed anger and disruptions in the mother-child relationship were the cause of IBD and of increased disease severity (Engel, 1958). Conclusions from these data, however, are limited due to the small number of patients enrolled, retrospective reporting, lack of control groups, and selection criteria (i.e., use of patients referred for psychotherapy). A more complicated multidetermined illness model has replaced this cause and effect model with studies documenting that psychological problems could *result* from having IBD and from having to deal with the complicated demands of the illness. Depression was recognized as a possible *reaction* to the stress and disruptions of living with IBD (Drossman, Patrick, Mitchell & Zagami, 1989). Burke, Meyer, Kochoshis, Orenstein, and Sauer (1989) reported that obsessive-compulsive symptoms in pediatric patients with IBD were likely to be *secondary* to the demands of dealing with IBD.

Current theories propose that psychological factors have little to do with the origins of IBD (Benkov & Winter, 1996; Levenstein, 1996). Although psychological factors may impact the course of the illness, the exact mechanism between the immune system, stress, and flare-ups of IBD has not been identified. Stress may affect a patient's ability to cope with IBD rather than cause the exacerbation of symptoms. The results of studies by Gerson, Schoholtz, Grega, and Barr (1998) are consistent with the findings of North, Alpers, Helzer, Spitznagel, & Clouse (1991), and Weitersheim, Kohler, and Feiereis (1992): patient life event stresses do not correlate with symptomatic exacerbation of IBD or the beginning of a relapse.

Gerson et al. (1998) suggest that stress may affect a patient's psychological ability to cope with his or her illness, rather than be directly responsible for an exacerbation of symptoms. In a recent study evaluating everyday stress and Crohn's disease activity, a time series analysis was conducted. In 55% of the cases, a significant correlation between daily hassles and disease activity was found. Patients whose symptomatology responded to stress did not differ from nonresponders in age, duration of the disease, disease activity, frequency of abdominal surgery, partnership situation, or statements concerning their average level of daily hassles. There was no confirmation of the assumption that daily hassles influence the symptomatology of the disease (Trane & Kosarz, 2000).

Despite a lack of data to support the etiological effects of psychological factors in relationship to IBD, a high percentage of patients with IBD (53% to 59%) are convinced that stress or their own personality is the principal cause of their IBD, while 90% believe it affects the disease course (Levenstein, 1996). Drossman (1988) analyzed physician beliefs regarding the etiology of IBD using a mail-in survey. Results indicated that physicians agreed that psychosocial factors did not contribute to the etiology or pathogenesis of IBD but did contribute to the clinical exacerbation of symptoms (more so in UC than in CD). Older physicians placed more importance on psychosocial factors in the etiology pathogenesis and exacerbation of these disorders than did younger physicians.

PROGNOSIS

For most children, the disease course of IBD is one of unpredictable exacerbation and remission. In children diagnosed with UC, 70% diagnosed will enter remission within 3 months following initial therapy, and approximately 50% will remain in remission over the next year. Colectomy within 5 years is required in up to 26% of children presenting with severe disease compared with 10% of those who have mild disease. Children who present with proctitis have up to a 70% likelihood of developing more extensive disease over time (Ballinger, 2000).

About 40% to 50% of patients with Crohn's disease will relapse in the first year after induction of disease remission (Ballinger, 2000). Only 1% of patients who have well-documented CD do not have at least one relapse after initial diagnosis. The risk of cancer is markedly increased for patients with long-standing ulcerative colitis. Surveillance colonoscopy and biopsy every 1 to 2 years is recommended for patients with UC for more than 7 years and disease beyond the splenic flexure. Patients with long-standing colonic CD have been reported to have a colon cancer risk similar to UC patients. The two most critical risk factors for adenocarcinoma are similar to duration of colitis (especially > 10 years) and extent of the colitis (pancolitis > left-sided colitis > proctitus) (Hyams, 2000).

Medical Aspects: Assessment and Treatment

Clinical Features

Kirschner (1998) identifies the following special aspects of the presentation of IBD in children and adolescents: delay in diagnosis, intestinal symptoms, and extraintestinal signs. Poor growth and delayed sexual maturation may dominate the early clinical picture, and they are important benchmarks. Mamula et al. (2003) cite the effect on growth and development as a particular aspect of pediatric IBD for which there is no adult equivalent. Growth delay in children with IBD is hypothesized to be secondary to inflammation, nutrient malabsorption, and undernutrition (Pappa, 2004). The combination of decreased intake and increased metabolic demands present an especially large burden for the body of a child or adolescent diagnosed with IBD. By the time most children are diagnosed with IBD, they are already somewhat malnourished. When IBD is active during critical periods of growth, it is extremely difficult to compensate for the increased demands with oral intake alone.

In addition to growth failure, abdominal pain, bloody diarrhea, fever, and weight loss are the most common physical manifestations in children and adolescents with IBD. Children and adolescents with IBD also present with significant extra intestinal symptoms, which vary in presentation from case to case. Up to 35% of pediatric IBD patients have at least one extra intestinal manifestation as a presenting sign (Mamula et al., 2003). Common extra intestinal symptoms include: mouth sores, back pain, erythema nosodum, pyoderma gangrenosum, and joint complaints. Anemia is also seen, secondarily to blood loss or poor nutrition.

Abnormalities in linear growth are a common presenting sign of CD. Decreased height velocity was shown to antedate the onset of CD in 88% of adolescents at one tertiary center. A fall in height velocity may also be the first indication of disease relapse and may be accompanied by only minor GI symptoms (Ballinger, 2000). Growth failure complicates the clinical course of children with IBD, more often in CD than in UC.

Patients diagnosed with UC generally present with bloody diarrhea, rectal bleeding, but little evidence for systemic disease. Typically a diagnosis is made with 6 months from the onset of the symptoms (Cuffari & Darbari, 2002). Diarrhea, occasionally bloody, is seen in 50% of patients who have CD. Perirectal inflammation with fissures and fistula occurs in about 25% of CD patients. Fever occurs in UC only in the presence of fulminant disease; whereas in CD, fever may occur in the absence of severe gastrointestinal symptoms and be diagnosed initially as a fever of unknown origin (Hyams, 2000). Abdominal pain is a more prominent problem among those who have CD. Abdominal pain in patients with UC is usually limited to the predefecatory period.

Evaluation

The diagnosis of IBD includes integration of information from (a) stool examinations; (b) blood tests; (c) radiological procedures (upper and lower gastrointestinal [GI] studies, computed tomography scans, and abdominal ultrasounds); and (d) endoscopic procedures (e.g., sigmoidoscopy, colonoscopy, and upper GI endoscopy). Endoscopy with biopsy is critical for confirming an IBD diagnosis.

Recently, with the purpose of aiding in multicenter, multinational collaboration, specific work-up procedures were established as the Porto Diagnostic criteria (ESPGHAN, 2005). To make a diagnosis of IBD, the following procedures are recommended: (1) a complete diagnostic program consisting of colonoscopy with ileal intubation; (2) upper GI endoscopy; (3) in all cases except definitive diagnosis of UC, radiologic contrast imaging of the small bowel; and (4) multiple biopsies from all segments of the GI tract are needed for a complete histologic evaluation. A diagnosis of IC cannot be made unless a full diagnosis program has been performed (ESPGHAN, 2005). Although fiber optic ileocolonoscopy with multiple mucosal biopsies coupled with quality barium studies has led to speedier and more accurate diagnoses (Walker-Smith, 2000), delay in diagnosis of IBD in the pediatric population continues to be a concern. The mean delay for the diagnosis of CD in children is reported to be between 7 to 11 months, in UC between 5 to 8 months, and in IC 14 months (Mamula et al., 2003). The delay in the diagnosis of CD appears to be prolonged if the disease affects more proximal bowel and if presenting symptoms do not include diarrhea.

The range of presenting signs and symptoms of IBD in children and adolescents is broad and often subtle. The diagnosis is particularly difficult when the presenting symptoms are uncharacteristic and consist mainly of extraintestinal manifestations (e.g., anorexia, back pain, anemia, fatigue, and joint complaints) (Mamula et al., 2003).

Treatment

The general goals of treatment for children and adolescents with IBD are to:

1. Achieve the best control of the inflammatory process with the least possible side effects from medication.
2. Promote growth through adequate nutrition.
3. Facilitate the patient's normal functioning (e.g., school attendance, peer contacts, involvement in sports). (Baldassano & Piccoli, 1999)

Treatment of pediatric and adolescent patients with IBD requires attention to issues unique to these age groups. In addition to intestinal symptoms, the treatment should involve nutritional support and control of extraintestinal manifestations and psychosocial well-being (Escher et al., 2003). The variability in the age of onset, sites of intestinal involvement, severity of intestinal disease, and extraintestinal manifestations, result in a broad range of clinical presentations that necessitate individualized therapy (Kirschner, 1995).

Drossman (1989) recommends the following steps for physicians treating patients with IBD: establish a therapeutic relationship, help the patient learn about IBD, involve the family, consider behavioral interventions, help the patient to avoid adopting a "sick role," and obtain psychiatric consultations when appropriate.

The medical management of IBD in children and adolescents is not standardized; it can include medical, nutritional, and surgical interventions.

The goal of medical therapy is to control symptoms, induce and maintain remission, prevent complications, and improve growth. The scarcity of clinical trials in the treatment of pediatric and adolescent patients with IBD has required the extrapolation from adult studies particularly in the management of aggressive or resistant disease (Pappa, 2004).

Disease remission and relapse prevention are the goals of pharmacological intervention. Specific pharmacological management depends of the level of disease activity. Effective pharmacological strategies are available for acute treatment of active CD, but long-term management remains problematic in many patients (Buller, 2001). Pharmacological therapy includes the use of the following medications: corticosteroids, 5-amino salicylic acid preparations, 6-mercaptopurine, cyclosporine, antibiotics (Metronidazole), and biological agents (infliximab). Steroids are indicated when there is acute disease that is unresponsive to other medications. In addition to coshingnoid features, weight gain, acne, and striae, the side effects of long-term use of steroids are significant and can include: growth suppression, cataracts, glaucoma, osteoporosis, hypertension (King, 2003), and avascular necrosis (Shapiro, Rothstein, Newman, Fletcher, & Halpin, 1985). For adolescents, the cosmetic side effects (e.g., acne, cushingoid features, weight gain, hirsutism, and striae) are particularly difficult affecting the quality of life of some patients, which can offset the potential physical benefit they provide. Researchers have developed new biologic therapies that target specific areas in the inflammatory process as opposed to the broad-based immunosuppressive approach of some older medications. Recent use of Remicade (infliximab) has shown encouraging results in the pediatric population (Kugathasan et al., 2002). A study evaluating short- and long-term efficacy of infliximab in children with UC showed a short-term response. Although the long-term response was lower, inflixmab did allow for the avoidance of a colectomy during the follow-up period (Eidelwein, Cuffari, Abadom, & Oliva-Hemker, 2005). Although immunosuppressants provide protection from relapse with long-term use and allow steroid sparing, the risk for potentially hazardous side effects requires careful consideration in pediatric patients (Buller, 2001).

By the time most children are diagnosed with IBD, they are already malnourished to some degree (Mamula, Markowitz, & Baldassano, 2003). The goals of nutritional therapy are to correct nutritional deficiencies due to reduced appetite, poor absorption, and diarrhea and to promote catch-up growth. Nutritional therapy can include: (a) dietary modification; (b) nutritional supplementation; and (c) total parenteral nutrition (TPN) therapy (Heuschkel, Menache, Megarian & Baird, 2000). Nutritional therapy can be supplemental or the primary therapy. There are no scientific data to support the efficacy of alternative diets or supplements. Another important reflection of overall nutritional status is progression of sexual development. Delay in the onset of pubertal development is common among adolescents with IBD, and active disease can potentially delay the onset of puberty indefinitely or slow down or arrest its progression. These potential effects have important psychosocial implications for the adolescent patient.

In addition to inducing and maintaining disease remission with minimal side effects, good symptom control, and an optimal health-related quality of life (HRQOL), disease control must be sufficient to facilitate normal growth and pubertal development (Bremner & Beattie, 2002). Complete bowel rest with parenteral nutritional support is associated with clinical improvement in 40% to 90% of patients with severe CD. Enteral nutrition is an important part of the primary therapy for active CD in patients for whom steroids are potentially harmful (i.e., children) and it is recommended as an adjunctive therapy for steroid-refractory and particularly steroid dependent CD patients (Hyams, 2002).

Surgical treatment is necessary when (a) medication cannot control the symptoms; (b) there is an intestinal obstruction; or (c) there are other complications. More than a third of people with child onset IBD will require surgery to manage the disease within 20 years of diagnosis (Langholz, Munkholm, Krasilnikoff, & Binder, 1998). Surgery for patients with UC is curative and it is now standard to perform sphincter-saving operations in patients with UC in whom medical therapy has been unsuccessful or accompanied by complications (Pappa, 2004). New techniques have been developed to avoid an ileostomy by creating an internal pouch from the small bowel and attaching it to the anal sphincter muscle. In comparison to adults, there is an increased prevalence of pouchitis after surgery in pediatric patients (Pappa, 2004).

The need for, and the timing of, colectomy in children is determined by weighing the response to medical therapy, risks of growth impairment, and ultimate cancer risk on one hand against the prospects of surgical cure, along with potential adverse effects after surgery.

In CD, the inflamed part of the intestine is removed (resection) and the two ends of the healthy bowel are joined together (anastomoses). This surgery may provide symptom-free years; however, it is not curative because the disease can recur in other parts of the intestinal tract. In addition, there is recurrence of histologic disease in surgical anastomosis that makes medication after surgery necessary to prevent recurrences.

Psychosocial Aspects: Patient and Family Concerns, Assessment, Treatment, and Clinical Features

Patient Concerns

The first author's experience has shown that discussion of the following issues can help to relieve patient concerns:

1. The unknown etiology of IBD.
2. The unpredictable course of the illness.
3. Embarrassment due to bathroom-related symptoms.
4. Fear of painful tests and procedures.
5. Treatment-related stresses such as: medication side-effects, restricted diets, and noncompliance struggles.

The lack of a known etiology and the unpredictable course of IBD are distressing both to patients and family members. The reality that compliance with the treatment regimen does not prevent a recurrence is anxiety producing, particularly with adolescents and young adults who are beginning to make future-oriented decisions. One of the most difficult aspects of having IBD is the embarrassment associated with bathroom-related symptoms. Children and adolescents are self-conscious about having to leave the classroom to use the bathroom because it calls attention to them. In addition, many school bathrooms do not have stall doors so there is no privacy. Anecdotal reports indicate that students stay home from school because of this issue (Cunningham, 2001). An increased prevalence of depression has been documented in children with CD (Engström, 1999; Rabbett et al., 1996; Burke, Meyer, Kochoshis, Orenstein, & Sauer, 1990).

Family Concerns

The following concerns are important to discuss with the patient's family:

1. Fear that IBD could lead to cancer in their children.
2. Fears that their children will be teased at school because of the side effects of the medication.
3. Problems due to growth retardation.
4. Concerns that IBD would affect fertility, conception, and pregnancy.
5. Awareness of the impact of IBD on the entire family, especially siblings.
6. Fears regarding future insurance problems.
7. Concerns about emotional impact of dealing with IBD.

The diagnosis of a child with a chronic illness such as IBD can cause stress on parents and the entire family (Drotar, 1981). Specific parental concerns, including noncompliance of teenagers with medication and diet, understanding the impact of IBD on the entire family, and school-related issues were found in groups created to identify the specific stressors for parents of pediatric patients with IBD and to simultaneously decrease parental anxiety (Cunningham, 2002). Parents reported that the group experience was helpful in decreasing their anxiety by the sharing of common experiences.

In 2001, at "Breaking the Silence about IBD," a seminar sponsored by the Crohn's and Colitis Foundation of America, parents of pediatric IBD patients identified the following illness-related concerns for their children: (a) fears that IBD could lead to cancer; (b) upset over their children being teased because of medication side effects; (c) problems related to growth retardation; (d) concerns about the effects of IBD on fertility, conception, and pregnancy; (e) awareness of impact of IBD on the entire family, including siblings; and (f) fears regarding insurance difficulties.

Health-Related Quality of Life Studies

Current psychosocial research related to pediatric and adolescent patients with IBD is focused on the impact of IBD on everyday life. Physicians have realized that traditional methods of evaluating the clinical status of patients with IBD may not accurately reflect how patients feel about their illness, how they function on a day-to-day basis, and ease their worries and concerns (Drossman et al., 1989). HRQOL studies of pediatric and adolescent patients with IBD have examined their psychological functioning, their academic and social functioning, and their family's functioning (Griffiths et al., 1999; Loonen, Grootenhuis, Last, Koopman, & Derkx, 2004; Loonen, Grootenhuis, Last, Koopman, & Derkx; 2002; Cunningham, Drotar, Palermo, McGowan, & Arendt, 2006).

Psychological Functioning

IBD in children and adolescents is often associated with depression, anxiety, and lowered self-esteem. Engström (1992) compared children with IBD, diabetes, and tension headaches to a control group of healthy children. In comparison to healthy controls and children with diabetes, patients with IBD had more depressive and anxiety disorders, were more pessimistic about the future, and had more difficulty discussing the illness. Moody, Eaden, and Mayberry (1999) reported that children with CD expressed fears and anxieties about their future and fears about participating in everyday childhood activities such as playing with friends, staying overnight at a friend's house, and going on vacation. Akobeng et al. (1999) found that children taking steroids exhibited more depressive symptoms then those patients with IBD who were not taking steroids. Helpful factors common to those patients doing well included (a) having knowledge about IBD, (b) open family communication, (c) social support network, and (d) someone with whom they could specifically discuss illness-related questions.

Social and Academic Functioning

Studies document significant social and academic morbidity of pediatric and adolescent patients with IBD. In comparison to healthy children, Akobeng et al. (1999) found that children with Crohn's disease missed more school and participated less in sports and peer-related activities. Ferguson, Sedgwick, and Drummond (1994) reported significant social morbidity in young adults with juvenile onset IBD reflected by: (a) absences from school; (b) interference with examinations; and (c) difficulties in pursuit of higher education. Moody et al. (1999) found that 66% of patients with IBD ages 6 to17 years had significant absences from school and 80% felt that they had underachieved on their examination due to their ill health. Patient responses also indicated that 67% reported a decrease in sports related activities, and 50% reported being unable to play with friends because of their illness. Lack of knowledge about IBD by teachers has been documented (Mayberry, 1999; Moody et al., 1999), as has the lack of information about the effects of IBD on the educational process. MacPhee, Hoffenberg, and Feranchak (1988) reported that adolescent patients with IBD were more likely to rely on family support networks for emotional support as opposed to their peers, suggesting a possible developmental lag.

Family Functioning

The significant effect on the family of having a child with IBD has been reported in a number of studies (Akobeng et al., 1999; Engström, 1992; Miller, 1997). Miller (1997) reported that 65% of parents worried about future issues and 55% worried if their children had problems at school. Parents reported that their lives had changed due to a decrease in social activities and changes in financial resources, particularly if one parent needed to stay home to care for the child. Poorer family functioning appears to be related to increased disease severity (Mackner, Sisson, & Crandall, 2004). Akobeng et al. (1999) have documented that families of children with IBD experience many difficulties that impact their lives.

Studies have also documented that siblings of patients with IBD are affected by the illness. Akobeng et al. (1999) found that healthy siblings of IBD patients were concerned about their parents keeping them uninformed about the illness. Engström (1999) found no increase in psychopathology of siblings with IBD, but he did find a decrease in their self-esteem and their self-reliance. Miller reported that siblings were worried about "being kept in the dark," their sibling being teased at school, and concerns that their sibling would have to go to the hospital. They also reported jealousy because of the special treatment and attention their sibling received. Healthy siblings of children and adolescents are also affected by the presence of IBD in the family. Engström (1992) found that in comparison to siblings of healthy children, siblings of patients with IBD had poorer peer relationships and had a tendency toward depression. In an earlier study, Wood et al. (1988) reported that CD siblings had more psychological disorders than UC siblings.

Past studies that evaluated the importance of HRQOL of pediatric and adolescents with IBD were limited due to lack of control groups, small sample sizes, use of focus groups, and the use of nonvalidated questionnaires. Two recent studies have addressed these methodological issues using both a validated measure of quality of life and a disease specific measure. Loonen, Grootenhuis, Last, Koopman, and Derkx (2002) studied the HRQOL of pediatric patients using both a generic and a disease-specific questionnaire. The authors, in an international collaboration, developed the Impact II and it has proven to be a well-validated instrument for discriminating between patients with varying disease activity states on all domains. The results reported that adolescent patients, especially those with CD, were severely affected in their HRQOL on four domains compared with their healthy peers. Impairment on motor functioning and autonomy was perceived as a threat to gaining independence from caregivers, and a high occurrence of negative emotions places patients at risk for depressive and behavioral disorders. In a study describing the association between coping styles and HRQOL of adolescents with IBD, Loonen, Grootenhuis, Last, and Derkx (2004) reported that adolescents with IBD use more avoidant coping styles than their healthy peers. Adolescents using a more predictive coping style (having positive expectations about the disease) and less use of a depressive reaction pattern are associated with better HRQOL in three out of six HRQOL domains.

DeBoer, Grootenhuis, Derkx, and Last (2005) found that, based on parent report, adolescents with IBD demonstrated worse HRQOL than the reference sample of healthy peers. However, Loonen and colleagues and DeBoer et al.'s (2005) findings were limited by two methodological problems: (1) the use of a historical control group based on a standardization sample of healthy children rather than children who were drawn from a population of similar demographics as the IBD sample; and (2) the failure to evaluate the impact of clinically relevant symptoms of IBD and treatments such as steroids on the HRQOL of children and adolescents with IBD.

Cunningham, Drotar, Palermo, McGowan & Arendt (2006), using a controlled group matched for age, sex and race, used validated HRQOL measures, and a disease-specific measure (Harvey & Bradshaw, 1980) found that children and adolescents with IBD demonstrated a lower HRQOL in comparison to healthy controls.

TABLE 3.2. Questions for Psychological Assessment of Pediatric and Adolescent Patients with IBD

A. Patient's Functioning

1. *Cognitive perceptions of IBD*. What is the child/teen's medical understanding of IBD? Of the cause of IBD? Do they understand the proposed treatment regimen; including possible side effects of the medications? What are their biggest fears about having IBD? Do they think that IBD is life threatening?

2. *Social functioning*. Are their friends aware of their IBD? Are they involved in any school-related or extracurricular activities? How does their illness interfere with socializing with their peers? What activities do they *not* participate in because of having IBD?

3. *School*. Has the child missed school days or had to repeat a grade because of IBD? Can they participate in a full academic schedule? Is there academic pressure because of missed school days? Is the school cooperative of special needs (e.g., bathroom privileges, the need for medicine)?

4. *Family relationships*. Is the family supportive? Who is responsible for making sure medication is taken? Do parents nag about diet and medication issues? Have parents become overprotective? What are the reactions of siblings and grandparents?

B. Assessment of the Family

1. Administer the Child Behavior Checklist (Achenbach, 1991) to primary care giver(s).

2. Determine the family's knowledge of IBD? What do they think is the cause of IBD? What are the strengths and the difficulties in the family system? Who manages patient care e.g., doctor's appointments, diet, medication? What are the stresses in the family system e.g., a sibling, grandparents due to patient's IBD?

Assessment

Psychosocial assessment should evaluate both the patient's functioning and the family's functioning. The characteristics of the child need to be assessed. These include: developmental functioning, coping skills, personality dynamics, hopes, fear, and how the child understands his or her body. As with any chronic illness, a child's developmental level plays a significant part in his or her understanding of and coping with IBD. Age-related assessments are necessary because of the developmental changes of the child over time. School-age children focus on immediate issues: pain due to shots, blood tests, and invasive procedures. They worry about nausea or having to use a public washroom. Restrictions around diet at school and social events cause discouragement and anger. Adolescent issues such as the need to be in control, peer pressure to conform, and body image concerns are significantly affected by IBD. Concerns regarding changes in appearance (e.g., weight gain, growth retardation, cushingoid features) are a major concern, as are functional and social limitations.

The questions presented in Table 3.2 can be used as a framework for the psychological assessment of pediatric and adolescent patients with IBD. Age-related assessments are necessary because of the developmental changes of the child over time.

Psychological Treatment: Strategic Points for Psychological Intervention with Pediatric and Adolescent Patients with IBD

At Diagnosis

Psychological intervention at the time of diagnosis focuses on acknowledging the patient's relief that a physical problem has been identified, providing information, and supporting the patient. Many pediatric patients have had little experience with disease, and the diagnosis of a chronic illness that needs long-term therapy requires a period of adjustment. Although IBD patients must deal with the reality that they have a chronic illness, the diagnosis of IBD can be a relief for some patients because their symptoms had been misattributed to psychological diagnoses such as depression, anorexia, chronic fatigue syndrome, or IBS. Education is an essential tool for coping with a difficult situation such as the new diagnosis of IBD in a child. Reports indicate that the quality of the initial educational process may impact subsequent outcome compliance and patient/family quality-of-life aspects. Day, Whitten, and Bohane (2005) determined that information distribution is vital in the management of children with chronic GI conditions such as IBD, and they advocate for educational activities as one of the essential roles of an IBD clinic. Many families had not even heard of IBD prior to their child's diagnosis, and the provision of information is important at diagnosis. To address this need, an "IBD library" was created to present information in innovative ways to patients and families. The library consists of patient-created books, videotapes of interviews with patients with IBD, and a listing of relevant websites. Feedback from patients, families, and medical staff indicates that this library has been helpful (Cunningham, 2001). Additional information of relevant websites is shared with patients and families (see p. 51).

In addition to education, support is needed for patients dealing with the extraordinary demands of medical care that IBD can require, including naso-gastric tubes, not being able to eat for long periods of time, and diagnostic procedures such as colonoscopies, barium enemas, and multiple X-rays. Patients with IBD may feel discouraged that their lives have been seriously abruptly and replaced by periods of intense pain, doctor's visits, blood tests, school pressures, and isolation from friends. Teenagers are often hesitant to discuss bowel function and there is the need to obtain information about stool pattern and frequency in a sensitive manner.

At Recurrence

A recurrence highlights one of the most stressful aspects of having IBD: the unpredictable course of the illness. Patients with IBD can do well for long periods of time and then become symptomatic with no apparent precipitant. A reoccurrence is devastating psychologically, stimulating intense feelings of depression, frustration, and fear. For some patients, a reoccurrence is the point at which they realize they have a chronic illness. Psychological inter-ventions should focus on helping patients identify and express their fears and their feelings of powerlessness. For most patients, the most difficult aspect of a flare-up is accepting the reality of having to restart intensive medical treat-ment, particularly with steroids.

It is important to elicit the child's or the adolescent's cognitive under-standing of his or her illness and why he or she had a reoccurrence (Perrin & Gerrity, 1984). Some patients worry that a reoccurrence means the inevitabil-ity of cancer or the need for a colostomy. Patients' fears may not be shared with their parents or with their gastroenterologists, and they silently live with misinformation and anxiety.

Treatment-Related Issues

Treatment-related problems include: medication side effects, diet restrictions, and family stress due to noncompliance problems, and the increased demands on the family. Some adolescents report that they would rather deal with the pain of the illness than with the treatment regimen, particularly the cosmetic side effects of the steroids.

Problems associated with the cosmetic side effects of the steroids, which can include cushingoid features, weight gain, acne, stretch marks, and mood swings, may be as difficult, if not worse, than the actual illness for most patients with IBD. To avoid the side effects of using steroids, adolescents, in particular, often minimize their symptoms until the pain becomes overwhelming and they cannot be ignored. Adherence to the medical treatment for patients with IBD seems to follow a predictable pattern in our practice. Immediately following the diagnosis of IBD, adherence is generally good. Many patients become increasingly noncompliant when they no longer feel sick, and they do not want to experience the medication side effects. To avoid the side effects, many adolescents stop taking their medicine without informing the medical staff, lower their dosage, or use the medication only reactively, such as when bleeding occurs. The danger of abruptly stopping the steroids must be explained to and reinforced with patients and families so as to avoid potential medical emergencies.

Noncompliance is a complicated issue and psychological intervention should involve the caregiver as well as the patient (La Greca & Schuman, 1995). Patients who are cooperative and productive in many areas of their lives may be deceptive regarding their IBD medication. Specific areas of noncompliance should be identified since patients with IBD can be compliant with dietary restrictions or moderating activity level and be noncompliant in another area, such as taking medication. Poor compliance with orally administered medication or failure to adhere to developing regimens for parentally administered drugs can adversely affect the natural history of CD (Hyams, & Markowitz, 2005). Many parents struggle with finding the balance between vigilance and intrusiveness. If noncompliance is a concern, our experience suggests that the monitoring of medication and diet is important. Future studies that develop strategies between the care provider and the patient to minimize deviation from the planned treatment regimen are particularly critical for children and adolescents.

School-Related Problems

School can pose many problems for patients with IBD. Patients with IBD need to use the bathroom more than other children and are often embarrassed to ask the teacher or obtain special permission. Children and adolescents are often teased at school about their appearance, especially cushingnoid features due to the steroid side effects. They may be singled out because they cannot participate in gym or other activities. Absenteeism has been identified as a problem for patients with IBD (Akobeng et al., 1999). School avoidance can become a problem due to abdominal pain, fatigue, increased frequency of bathroom use, and peer teasing so the child or adolescent with IBD should be encouraged to attend school, even part time. Moody et al. (1999) used a validated questionnaire to assess issues for children and found that many of their teachers knew very little about Crohn's disease. Parents are encouraged to establish a 504 Plan at school, which identifies IBD as a medical problem. This plan can formalize school strategies, such as bathroom usage, that are helpful to the patient. A 504 Plan is also a unique opportunity to educate school personnel about IBD. Brochures from the Crohn's and Colitis Foundation of America (CCFA) specifically designed for teachers are helpful (http://www.ccfa.org).

GUIDELINES FOR PSYCHOSOCIAL INTERVENTION

The following guidelines have been found to be helpful for psychosocial intervention with pediatric and adolescent patients with IBD.

1. Be knowledgeable about the medical aspects of IBD: the presenting symptoms, the diagnostic procedures, the treatment modalities, and the medication side effects. Knowledge of these issues is critical to: (a) understand what the patient is experiencing, (b) to not misinterpret disease symptoms such as fatigue or anorexia, and (c) to enhance dialogue with pediatric gastroenterologists.
2. Ideally, the introduction of the pediatric psychologist should occur at the time of diagnosis or as early in the disease course as possible, since a primary prevention approach that includes education, anticipatory guidance, and multidisciplinary involvement is most effective.
3. Elicit the patient's and the family's knowledge of IBD in order to clarify misconceptions about the illness prognosis and misattributions regarding etiology. Provide families with information about local resources such as the Crohn's and Colitis Foundation of America. See websites that may be helpful.
4. Normalize reactions to dealing with IBD and the treatment regimen for the patient and the family. Knowing that their fears about bathroom issues or about medication side effects are common for patients with IBD may help to decrease their anxiety.
5. Teach patients and families skills to cope with their illness. For patients, these skills might include relaxation techniques or cognitive strategies to cope with their negative cognitions about appearance. For parents, general parenting techniques, suggestions regarding medication compliance, and emotional support on an individual basis or in the context of a parent support group are helpful.

NEW DIRECTIONS: CLINICAL CARE AND RESEARCH

Health care transition has become an issue of increasing concern and the American Academy of Pediatrics has made health care transition one of its priorities in an effort to ensure comprehensive community-based service for all children and youth with special needs. Transitioning patients from a pediatric clinic to an adult gastroenterology clinic could result in improved compliance with therapy and effective planning of long-range life needs. Such programs could also address the needs for a benefits package to be designed covering issues of continuing health insurance, life insurance, and disability (Mamula & Markowitz, 2003).

The importance of multidisciplinary care for pediatric and adolescent patients with IBD has been recognized through research (Wood et al., 1987; King, 2003; Mackner, 2004; Engström, 1992) and clinically (Cunningham,

2001). However, the future of a comprehensive biopsychosocial approach to the treatment of children and adolescents with IBD is compromised by the current climate of managed care. Pediatric gastroenterologists and pediatric psychologists have time constraints that impact how they would "ideally" like to practice. Until studies can be done that empirically validate the benefits of psychosocial intervention, some pediatric and adolescent patients with IBD and their families may have psychological sequelae that may have been prevented.

To date, limitations due to methodological problems in the existing research in children and adolescents with IBD have affected the validity of the outcomes presented (Mackner, Sisson, & Crandall, 2004). Almost all of the current research in pediatric IBD is cross-sectional. Future studies need to address issues of sample size, use of randomized controlled trials, and clear disease-specific questionnaires, which have been normed and validated.

Specific areas of future investigation should examine the following issues:

1. There are few research studies in the pediatric literature that documents the benefit of psychotherapy, behavioral medicine techniques, or psychotropic medications to affect the long-term course of IBD in children and adolescents. Psychotherapy with adults has shown to increase the patient's sense of control and his or her ability to withstand the stress of dealing with IBD (Levenstein, 1996). A pilot study demonstrated that a manual-based CBT approach including a physical illness narrative, social skills enhancement, and family components is a safe, feasible, and promising approach to treat physically ill adolescents with depression. Use of the Primary and Secondary Control Enhancement Training (PASCET) manual improved adolescents' perceptions of their general health and physical functioning, although illness severity measures remained unchanged (Szigethy, Whjitton, Warren, DeMasso, & Weisz, 2004). Well-designed studies examining these issues would provide information that could have important clinical ramifications.

2. Since IBD is often diagnosed during adolescence, the effects of navigating through periods of developmental transitions with a diagnosis of IBD needs to be further studied. Issues related to self-esteem, employment, and delayed sexual development need to be examined. Mackner, Sisson, & Crandall (2004) propose a developmental perspective to investigate the process of adjustment to IBD and to identify risk factors for poor adjustment. As the incidence of IBD increases, particularly the overall incidence of CD and the incidence of CD in young children, clinical intervention that addresses psychosocial needs will become an important issue. Evidence-based research, which documents the importance of developmental issues, could provide a rich opportunity for anticipatory guidance to patients and families and the opportunity for a significant preventative mental health effect.

REFERENCES

Achenbach, T. (1991). Manual of the Child Behavior Checklist(CBCL). Burlington, VT: *University Associates of Psychiatry*.

Afzal, M. A., Armitage, E., Begley, J., Bentley, Minor, Ghosh, et al. (1998). Absence of detectable measles virus genome sequence in inflammatory bowel disease tissues and peripheral blood lymphocytes. *Journal of Medical Virology, 55*, 243–249.

Akobeng, A. K., Suresh-Babu, M. V., Firth, D., Miller, V., Mir, P., & Thomas, A. G. (1999). Quality of life in children with Crohn's disease: A pilot study. *Journal of Pediatric Gastroenterology and Nutrition, 4*, S37–39.

Auvin, S., Molinie, F., Gower-Rousseau, C., Brazier, F., Merle, V., Grandbastien, B., Marti, R., Lerebours, E., Dupas, J. L., Colombel, J. F., Salomez, J. L., Cortot, A., Turck, D. (2005). Incidence, clinical presentation and location at diagnosis of pediatric inflammatory bowel disease: A prospective population-based study in northern France (1988-1999). *Journal of Pediatric Gastroenterology and Nutrition, 41*(1), 49–55.

Baldassano, R. N., & Piccoli, D. A. (1999). Inflammatory bowel disease in pediatric and adolescent patients. *Gastroenterology Clinics of North America, 28*, 445–458.

Ballinger, A. B. (2000). Epidemiology, natural history and prognosis of inflammatory bowel disease. In D. Ramptan (Ed.), *Inflammatory bowel disease* (pp. 59–70). Martin Dunitz.

Banez, G., & Cunningham, C. (2003). Pediatric gastrointestinal disorders: Recurrent abdominal pain, inflammatory bowel disease, and rumination disorder/cyclic vomiting. In M. C. Roberts (Ed.), *Handbook of pediatric psychology, 3rd ed.* (pp. 462–478). New York: Guilford.

Baron, S., Turck, D., Leplat, C., Merle, V., Gower-Rousseau, C., Marti, R., Yzet, T., Lerebours, E., Dupas, J. L., Debeugny, S., Salomez, J. L., Cortot, A., & Colombel, J. F. (2005). Environmental risk factors in paediatric inflammatory bowel diseases: A population based case control study. *Gut, 54*(3), 357–363.

Benkov, K. J., & Winter, H. S. (1966). *Managing your child's Crohn's disease or ulcerative colitis.* New York: Master Media Limited.

Brant, S. R., Panhuysen, C. I. M., Bailey-Wilson, J. E. et al. (2000). Linkage heterogeneity for the IBD1 locus in Crohn's disease pedigrees by disease onset and severity. *Gastroenterology, 119*, 1483–1490.

Bremner, A. R., & Beattie, R. M. (2002). Theory of Crohn's disease in childhood. *Expert Opinions in Pharmacology, 3*(7), 809–825.

Buller, H. (2001). Objectives and outcomes in the conventional treatment of pediatric Crohn's disease. *Journal of Pediatric Gastroenterology and Nutrition, 33*(Suppl. 1), S11–S18.

Burke, P., Kocoshis, S. A., Chandra, R., Whiteway, M., & Sauer, J. (1990). Determinants of depression in recent onset pediatric inflammatory bowel disease. *Journal of the American Academy of Child and Adolesdent Psychiatry, 4*, 608–610.

Burke, P., Meyer, V., Kochoshis, S., Orenstein, D., & Sauer, J. (1989). Obsessive-compulsive symptoms in childhood inflammatory bowel disease and cystic fibrosis. *Journal of the American Academy of Child and Adolescent Psychiatry, 4*, 525–527.

Cuffari, C., & Darbari, A. (2002). Inflammatory bowel disease in the pediatric and adolescent patient. *Gastroenterology Clinics of North America, 31*, 275–291.

Cunningham, C. (2001). A unique educational intervention for pediatric and adolescent patients with IBD. Society of pediatric psychology. "Progress Notes" *25*(3), 4–5.

Cunningham, C. (2002). Talking with teens: A pediatric Crohn's disease and ulcervative colitis seminar. Independence, Ohio.

Cunningham, C., Drotar, D., Palermo, T., McGowan, K., Arendt, R. (2006). Health-Related Quality of Life in Children and Adolescents with Inflammatory Bowel Disease. Unpublished manuscript.

Day, A. S., Whitten, K. E., & Bohane, T. D. (2005). Childhood inflammatory bowel disease: Parental concerns and expectations. *World Journal of Gasteroenterology, 11*(7), 1028–1031.

DeBoer, M., Grootenhuis, M., Derkx, B., & Last, B. (2005). Health-related quality of life and psychosocial functioning of adolescents with inflammatory bowel disease. *Inflammatory Bowel Disease, 11*(4) 400–406.

Drossman, D. A. (2000). The functional gastrointestinal disorders and the Rome II process. In
    D. A. Drossman, E. Corazziari, N. J. Talley, W. G. Thompson, & W. E. Whitehead (Eds.),
    Rome II: The functional gastrointestinal disorders (pp. 1–29). Lawrence, KS: Allen Press.
Drossman, D. A., Leserman, J., Mitchell, C. M., Li, Z. M., Zagami, E. A., & Patrick, D. L.
    (1991). Health status and health care use in person with inflammatory bowel disease.
    Digestive Diseases and Sciences, 36, 1746–1755.
Drossman, D. A., Patrick, D. L., Mitchell, C. M. et al. (1989). Health-related quality of inflam-
    matory bowel disease. Functional status and patient worries and concerns. *Digestive
    Diseases and Sciences, 34*, 1379–1386.
Drotar, D. (1981). Psychological perspectives in chronic childhood illness. *Journal of Pediatric
    Psychology, 6*(3), 211–228.
Eidelwein, A., Cuffari, C., Abadom, V., Oliva-Hemker, M. (2005, March). Infliximab efficacy in
    pediatric ulcerative colitis. *Inflammatory Bowel Disease, 11*(3), 213–218.
Engel, G. (1958). Studies of ulcerative colitis. Psychological aspects and their implications for
    treatment. *American Journal of Digestive Diseases, 4*, 315–337.
Engström, I. (1992). Mental health and psychological functioning in children and adolescents
    with inflammatory bowel disease: A comparison with children having other chronic ill-
    nesses and with healthy children. *Journal of Child Psychology and Psychiatry, 33*, 563–582.
Engström, I. (1999). Inflammatory bowel disease in children and adolescents: Mental health and
    family functioning. *Journal of Pediatric Gastroenterology and Nutrition, 28*(4), S28–S33.
Escher, J. C., Taminiau, J. A. J. M., Nieuwenhuis, E. E. S., Buller, H. A., & Grand, R. J. (2003).
    Treatment of inflammatory bowel disease in childhood: Best available evidence.
    Inflammatory Bowel Diseases, 9(1), 34–58.
Ferguson, A., Sedgwick, D. M., & Drummond, J. (1994). Morbidity of juvenile-onset inflammatory
    bowel disease: Effects on education and employment in early adult life. *Gut, 35*, 665–668.
Gerson, M.-J., Schoholtz, J., Grega, C. H., & Barr, D. R. (1998). The importance of the family
    content in inflammatory bowel disease. *Mount Sinai Journal of Medicine, 65*(5–6), 398–403.
Griffiths, A. M., Nicholas, D., Smith, C., Munk, M., Stephens, D., Durno, C. et al. (1999).
    Development of a quality-of-life index for pediatric inflammatory bowel disease: dealing
    with differences related to age and IBD type. *Journal of Pediatric Gastroenterology and
    Nutrition, 4*, S46–52.
Gryboski, J. D. (1994). Crohn's disease in children 10 years old and younger: Comparison with
    ulcerative colitis. *Journal of Pediatric Gastroenterology and Nutrition, 18*, 174–182.
Harvey, R. F., & Bradshaw, J. M. (1980). A simple index of Crohn's disease activity, *Lancet, 1*, 514.
Heuschkel, R. B., Menache, C. C., Megarian, J. T., & Baird, A. E. (2000). Enteral nutrition and
    corticosteroids in the treatment of acute Crohn's disease in children. *Journal of Pediatric
    Gastroenterology and Nutrition, 31*, 8–15.
Heyman, M. B., Kirschner, B. S., Gold, B. D., Ferry, G., Baldassano, R., Cohen, S. A., Winter,
    H. S., Fain, P., King, C., Smith, T., & El-Serag, H. B. (2005). Children with early-onset
    inflammatory bowel disease (IBD): Analysis of a pediatric IBD consortium registry.
    Journal of Pediatrics, 146(1), 35–40.
Hyams, J. S. (1996). Crohn's disease in children. *Pediatric Clinics of North America, 43*, 255–277.
Hyams, J. S. (2002). Diet and gastrointestinal disease. *Current Opinions in Pediatrics, 14*, 567–569.
Hyams, J. S., Burke, G., Davis, P. M., Rzepsaki, B., & Andrulonis, P. A. (1996). Abdominal pain
    and irritable bowel syndrome in adolescents: A community-based study. *Journal of
    Pediatrics, 129*, 220–226.
IBD Working Group of the European Society for Paediatric Gastroenterology, Hepatology, and
    Nutrition (ESPGHAN) (2005). Inflammatory bowel disease in children and adolescents:
    recommendations for diagnosis—the Porto criteria. *Journal of Pediatric Gastroenterology
    and Nutrition, 41*(1), 1–7.
Kanner, L. (1972). *Child psychiatry* (4th ed., pp. 463–464). Springfield, IL: Charles C. Thomas.
Kim S., & Ferry, G. (2002). Inflammatory bowel diseases in children. *Current Problems in
    Pediatric Adolescent Health Care, 32*, 108–132.
King, R. A. (2003). Pediatric inflammatory bowel disease. *Child Adolescent Psychiatric Clinics
    of North America, 12*, 967–995.

Kirschner, B. S. (1998). Differences in the management of inflammatory bowel disease in children and adolescents compared to adults. *Netherlands Journal of Medicine, 53*, S13–S18.

Korelitz, B. I. (1982). Epidemiological and psychosocial aspects of inflammatory bowel disease with observation on children, families, and pregnancy. *American Journal of Gastroenterology, 77*, 929–933.

Kugathasan, S., Judd, R. H., Hoffman, R. G., Heikenen, J., Telega, G., Khan, F. et al. (2003). Epidemiologic and clinical characteristics of children with newly diagnosed inflammatory bowel disease in Wisconsin: A statewide population-based study. *Journal of Pediatrics, 143*, 525–531.

Kugathasan, S., Levy, M. B., Saeian, K., Vasilopoulos, S., Kim, J. R., Prajapati, O. et al., (2002). Infliximab retreatment in adults and children with Crohn's disease: Risk factors for the development of delayed severe systemic reaction. *American Journal of Gastroenterology, 97*, 1408–1424.

La Greca, A. M., & Schuman, W. B. (1995). Adherence to prescribed medical regimens. In M. C. Roberts (Ed.), *Handbook of pediatric psychology* (pp. 55–83). New York: Guilford.

Langholz, E., Munkholm, P., Krasilnikoff, P. A., & Binder, V. (1997). Inflammatory bowel disease with onset in childhood. *Scandinavian Journal of Gastroenterology, 32*, 139–147.

Langholz, E., Munkholm, P., Krasilnikoff, P. A., & Binder, V. (1998). Inflammatory bowel diseases in children. *Ugeskrift for Laeger, 160*, 5648–5654.

Levenstien, S. (1996). Is there health in wellness? *Journal of Clinical Gastroenterology, 23*(2), 94–96.

Levenstein, S. (1996). Psychosocial issues in Crohn's disease. In C. Prantera & B. Korelitz, (Eds.), *Crohn's disease* (pp. 429–443). New York: Marcel Dekker.

Loonen, H. J., Grootenhuis, M. A., Last, B. F., & Derkx, H. H. F. (2004). Coping strategies and quality of life of adolescents with inflammatory bowel disease. *Quality of Life Research, 13*, 1011–1019.

Loonen, H. J., Grootenhuis, M. A., Last, B. F., Koopman, H. M., Derkx, H. H. F. (2002). Quality of Life in pediatric inflammatory bowel disease measured by a generic and disease-specific questionnaire. *Acta Paediatrica, 91*, 348–357.

Mackner, L. M., Sisson, D. P., Crandall,W. V. (2004). Psychosocial issues in pediatric IBD. *Journal of Pediatric Psychology, 29*(4), 243–257.

MacPhee, M., Hoffenberg, E. J., & Feranchak, A. (1988). Quality-of-life factors in adolescents inflammatory bowel disease. *Inflammatory Bowel Disorder, 1*, 6–11.

Mamula, P., Markowitz, J. E., Baldassano, R. N., (2003). *Gastroenterology Clinics of North America, 32*, 967–995.

Mayberry, J. F. (1999). Impact of inflammatory bowel disease on educational achievements and work prospects. *Journal of Pediatric Gastroenterology and Nutrition, 28*, S34–36.

Moody, G., Eaden, J., & Mayberry, J. (1999). Social implications of childhood Crohn's disease. *Journal of Pediatric Gastroenterology and Nutrition, 28*, S43–45.

North, C. S., Alpers, D. H., Helzer, J. E., Spitznagel, E. L., & Clouse, R. E. (1991). Do life events or depression exacerbate inflammatory bowel disease? A prospective study. *Annals of Internal Medicine, 114*, 381–386.

Pappa, H. M., Semrin, G., Walker, T. R., & Grand, R. J. (2004). Pediatric inflammatory bowel disease. *Current Opinion in Gastroenterology, 20*, 333–340.

Perrin, E. C., & Gerrity, P. S. (1984). Development of children with a chronic illness. *Pediatric Clinics of North America, 31*, 19–31.

Rabbett, H., Elbadri, A., Thwaites, R., Northover, H., Dady, I., Firth, D. et al. (1996). Quality-of-life in children with Crohn's disease. *Journal of Pediatric Gastroenterology and Nutrition, 5*, 528–533.

Rasquin-Weber, A., Hyman P. E., Cucchiara, S., Fleisher, D. R., Hyams, J. S., Milla, P. J. et al. (1999). Childhood functional gastrointestinal disorders. *Gut, 45*(Suppl. 2), I160–I168.

Rice, H. E., & Chuang, E. (1999). Current management of pediatric inflammatory bowel disease. *Seminars in Pediatric Surgery, 8*, 221–228.

Ronald, A., Bremner, F., & Beattie, R. M. (2002). Therapy of Crohn's disease in childhood. *Expert Opinions in Pharmacotherapy, 3*(7), 809–825.

Sachar, D. (1987). Crohn's disease: A family affair. *Gastroenterology, 111*(83), 813–825.

Shapiro, S. C., Rothstein, F. C., Newman, A. J., Fletcher, B., Halpin, & T. C. Jr. (1985) Multifocal osteonecrosis in adolescents with Crohn's disease: A complication of therapy? *Journal of Pediatric Gastroenterology and Nutrition, 4*(3)502–506.

Szigethy, E., Whjitton, S. W., Warren, A. L., DeMaso, D. R., & Weisz, J. (2004, December). Cognitive behavioral therapy for depression in adolescents with inflammatory bowel disease: A pilot study. *American Academy of Child and Adolescent Psychiatry*, 43: 12.

Trane, H. C., & Kosarz, P. (2000). Everyday stress and Crohn's disease activity: A time series analysis of 20 single cases. *International Journal of Behavioral Medicine, 6*(2), 101–119.

Walker-Smith, J. A. (2000). Chronic inflammatory bowel disease in children: a complex problem in management. *Postgraduate Medical Journal, 76,* 469–472.

Walker-Smith, J. A., & Sanderson, I. R. (1999). Diagnostic criteria for chronic inflammatory bowel disease in childhood. In B. R. Bistrian & J. A. Walker-Smith (Eds.), *Inflammatory bowel diseases,* Nestec Nutrition Workshop Series Clinical & Performance Programming (Vol. 2, pp. 107–120). Basel: Nestec Ltd., Vevey/S. Kerger AG.

Weinstein, T. A., Levine, M., Pettei, M. J., Gold, D. M., Kessler, B. H., & Levine, J. J. (2003). Age and family history at presentation of pediatric inflammatory bowel disease. *Journal of Pediatric Gasteroenterology and Nutrition, 37,* 609–618.

Weitersheim, J. V., Kohler, T., & Feiereis, H. (1992). Relapse-precipitating life events and feelings in patients with inflammatory bowel disease. *Psychotherapy and Psychosomatics, 58,* 103–112.

Whitehead, W. E., & Schuster, M. M. (1985). Rumination syndrome, vomiting, aerophagia, and belching. In W. E. Whitehead & M. M. Schuster (Eds.), *Gastrointestinal disorders: Behavioral and physiological basis for treatment* (pp. 67–90). Orlando, FL: Academic Press.

Wood, B., Watkins, J. B., Boyle, J. T., Noqueria, J., Zimand, E., & Carrol, L. (1987). Psychological functioning in children with Crohn's disease and ulcerative colitis: Implications for models of psychobiological interaction. *Journal of the American Academy of Child and Adolescent Psychiatry, 26,* 774–781.

WEBSITES

North American Society for Pediatric Gastroenterology, Hepatology, and Nutrition
PO Box 6
Flourtown, PA 19031
(215) 233-0808
www.naspgn.org

Crohn & Colitis Foundations of America
386 Park Avenue South
New York, NY 10016-8804
(800) 343-3637
www.ccfa.org

United Ostomy Association, Inc.
19772 MacArthur Boulevard, Suite 200
Irvine, CA 92612-2405
(800) 826-0826
www.uoa.org

Wound, Ostomy, and Continence Nurses Society
4700 West Lake Avenue
Glenview, IL 60025
(888) 224-WOCN (9626)
www.wocn.org

Esophageal Disorders | 4

ESOPHAGEAL FUNCTIONING

The esophagus is a strong, muscular hollow tube, which connects the mouth to the stomach, starting at the cricopharyngeal muscle to a point below the diaphragm where it joins the stomach. The esophagus has two major functions: to propel fluid or food from the mouth into the stomach and to prevent retrograde flow of gastric contents inbetween swallows. These two apparently simple tasks are accomplished by complex mechanisms (Vandenplas & Hassall, 2002). The esophagus is not involved in the absorption, storage, or the digestion of food. The esophagus is closed at the top by the upper esophageal sphincter (UES) and at the lower end by the lower esophageal sphincter (LES). The wall of the esophagus is composed of muscle; the upper third is striated muscle, the lower third is smooth muscle, and the middle portion is composed of a mixture of smooth and striated muscle (Whitehead & Schuster, 1985). These layers of muscle squeeze the food along by a wavelike motion known as peristalsis, which is controlled by the autonomic nervous system. The esophagus is no longer viewed as a passive transport tube, but rather as an organ that is an integral part of the gastrointestinal (GI) system (Figure 4.1).

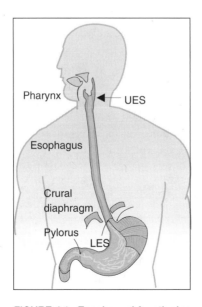

FIGURE 4.1. Esophageal functioning

ESOPHAGEAL DISORDERS

A range of physical problems occurring in the esophagus of pediatric and adolescent patients has been documented (Kumar & Sarvanthanan, 2003; Orenstein, Izadnia, & Khan, 1999; Vandenplas & Hegar, 2000). The recent increase in interest is due to a number of factors: (1) improved diagnostic technologies in areas such as pediatric endoscopy; (2) improved comprehension of the immunologic basis for inflammatory processes; and (3) a change in clinical opinion that recognizes that esophageal disease is a major cause of nonspecific symptoms such as infant colic, feeding disorders, and recurrent abdominal pain (Thompson, 2002).

Additionally, there has been an increased awareness of the complex interaction of causative factors that can lead to esophageal disorders. Interactions between the emotional state and esophageal functioning have also been noted repeatedly overtime (Deary, Wilson, & Kelly, 1995; Richter & Bradley, 1996). In 1893, Kronecker and Meltzer observed that esophageal contractions could be induced by "psychic upset." Since the late 1970s, interest in examining the relationships between psychosocial factors and esophageal diseases—particularly motility disorders—has increased.

The Rome II group defines functional esophageal disorders as disorders that represent chronic symptoms yet have no identifiable structural or metabolic basis (Clouse, Richter, Heading, Janseens, & Wilson, 1999). The functional esophageal disorders include globus and rumination syndrome, and symptoms that typify esophageal diseases are chest pain, heartburn, and dysphagia. Mechanisms responsible for the symptoms are poorly understood because of a combination of physiologic and psychosocial factors thought to be responsible for escalating symptoms to a level requiring medical attention (Clouse & Lustman, 1988). However, as with other GI disorders, the pathways that physiological, social, and psychophysiological factors interact with and influence the onset or the course of esophageal disorders are not definitively known. In children and adolescents, issues related to growth and development further impact these processes. This chapter will focus on esophageal disorders likely to occur in children and adolescents with attention to biopsychosocial factors. These include: globus sensation, gastroesophageal reflux—simple reflux (GER), gastroesophageal reflux disease (GERD), and esophageal motility disorders.

Globus Sensation

Swallowing

Swallowing is a complex, usually autonomic function that is divided into three phases: oral, pharyngeal, and esophageal. The mouth prepares the food for swallowing by chewing, lubrication, and the formation of a mound of food, which is then presented to the pharynx by the tongue. Protective mechanisms keep food out of the airway during pharyngeal transit. The peristaltic waves are initiated by swallowing. The relaxation and the opening of the UES direct the food into the esophagus. Esophageal peristalsis is coordinated with the pharyngeal contraction and the contraction of the UES to continue the propulsion of food toward the stomach. The LES relaxes nearly simultaneously with the UES to allow rapidly moving liquids to enter the stomach (Orenstein, 1997). The LES then contracts to prevent reflux of acidic stomach contents back into the esophagus. Motility between the upper and lower sphincter muscles in a typically functioning esophagus has been described as that of "exquisite coordination" (Herbst, 1996).

Definition of Condition

The globus symptom is a consistent clinical complaint, described by patients as "a lump in the throat," tightness, or a constriction, which results in considerable anxiety concerning choking (Bishop & Riley, 1988; Moloy & Charter, 1982). Globus is a sensory symptom that does not interfere with swallowing, but many patients experience mild change in deglutitive motor function just short of real swallowing problems (Wilson, 1992). The symptom is considered functional when no organic explanation is detected (Clouse, 1999). The globus sensation is easy to identify clinically, yet there is no consensus regarding a definition.

The Rome Group II defines the globus sensation as one occurring for at least 12 weeks which need not be consecutive, in the preceding 12 months of: (1) the persistent or intermittent sensation of a lump or foreign body in the throat; (2) occurrence of the sensation between meals; (3) absence of dysphagia and odynophagia; and (4) absence of pathologic gastroesophageal reflux, achalasia, or other motility disorders with a recognized pathologic basis (Clouse, 1999). The diagnostic criteria are the same for children and adolescents as for adults.

Early definitions of the globus sensation exist. Hippocrates described it as a disease of women attributed to "the wanderings of an untethered uterus." Psychoanalytically oriented clinicians from the 1930s to the present have defined the globus sensation as "globus hystericus," a type of conversion disorder. The term "globus hystericus" is controversial and viewed as "outdated" (Bradley & Narula, 1987). There is a lack of evidence-based support for globus as a conversion disorder; yet case studies citing "globus hystericus" are still published (Pehlivanturk & Unal, 2002). As recently as 2004, a review article defined the globus sensation as a "specific form of conversion disorder" (Finkenbine & Miele, 2004).

Culbert, Kajander, Kohen, and Reaney (1996) distinguished between disorders associated with the act of swallowing and disorders occurring exclusive of the act of swallowing in children. Their conceptualization includes disorders that are associated with the act of swallowing—organic dysphagia, developmental dysphagia, and functional dysphagia—and disorders that occur exclusive of swallowing including: globus hystericus, food aversion, phagophobia, and a hyperactive gag reflex. In addition, the conceptualization of Culbert, Kajander, Kohen, & Reaney (1996) includes the possibility that these phenomena can occur in varying combinations and sequences.

Clinical Presentation

Children's descriptions of the globus sensation vary considerably: they describe the sensation as "there is something stuck," "I can't swallow anything hard because I will choke," or "I feel a lump." The quality of the lump described can vary as can symptoms that are less precise, such as the feeling of the "throat closing off" or "a generalized choking sensation" (Deary, Wilson, Harris, & McDougall, 1995). Pain has also been described (Finkenbine & Miele, 2004). The globus sensation is often associated with dry swallowing or the need to dry swallow.

In the first author's practice, the presentation of the sensation globus is most common in younger children who have experienced a traumatic choking event. Physical sequelae from the globus sensation can include self-imposed dietary restrictions, which may interfere with adequate nutrition. Some children who report the globus sensation after an episode of choking will stop eating solid foods from one day to the next. Other children will gradually decrease the amount of food they eat. Many children will consume only liquids or a very soft diet including puddings and yogurts. Attempts to eat solids become rituals of chewing excessively to pulverize the food so that it is in liquid form when it is swallowed. Meals take a much longer time. There is a sense that the child would like to eat but is afraid. When pressured to eat, the child will become tearful and panicked. The level of frustration with eating and meals is increased for the patient and family members.

Psychosocial sequelae from the globus sensation can include limitations in the child's or adolescent's social life because of embarrassment over eating in front of others. Children will refuse snacks at school and they will not eat lunch at school because of their fear of choking or their embarrassment of the limited types of food that they are eating (e.g., puddings and gelatin). Restriction of daily activities including school can occur as well as increasing social isolation.

Epidemiology

There are few data regarding the incidence or the prevalence of globus sensation in children and adolescents. Varying opinions regarding the etiology of this symptom have contributed to this paucity of data: a discrepancy exists between those who define globus sensation as an uncommon conversion disorder (Finkenbine & Miele, 2004) and those who ascribe physical etiologies to the sensation (Herbst, 1996). One study reported that the globus sensation was the primary symptom of approximately 7% of children and adolescents diagnosed with conversion disorders (Steinhausen, Aster, Pfeiffer, & Gobel, 1989).

Course and Prognosis

There is little data or information regarding the course of the globus sensation in children and adolescents. In adults the globus sensation frequently recurs, which is attributed to the fact that the pathogenesis of this disorder, which can involve multiple factors, is unknown (Richter & Bradley, 1996).

Donahue, Thevenin, and Runyon (1997) reported in children that the symptoms of globus typically remit within 2 weeks. Nevertheless, if left untreated, the fear of choking and subsequent food refusal can lead to malnutrition, delayed development, and life-threatening weight loss (Bithony & Dubowitz, 1985). Factors that are associated with good prognosis for recovery include: early onset, supportive family members who are actively involved in treatment, and the lack of environmental and internal conflicts (Steinhausen, Aster, Pfeiffer, & Gobel, 1989).

Chatoor, Conley, and Dickson (1988) described the acute onset of anxiety about eating and the subsequent food refusal in children who either experienced or observed a severe choking episode. Factors that influenced the course and the severity of the disorders were the degree of preexisting psychopathology and the subsequent reaction of the family.

Etiology

Different theories have been proposed with respect to the etiology of globus sensation, most differentiating between organic and nonorganic causes (Moser et al., 1998). However, a simple dichotomous view (physical or psychological) of this symptom is insufficient (Engel, 1977; Richter & Bradley, 1996; Liebowitz, 1987). The etiology of the globus sensation has been reported as a symptom indicative of (1) a physical disorder such as GER, (2) a psychiatric disorder such as anxiety, (3) two simultaneously occurring disorders, one physical and one psychiatric, (4) the reaction to an experienced or an observed choking incident, and (5) a learned response to environmental factors.

Physical Explanation

Data for a physiologic explanation of globus sensation have produced conflicting results (Orenstein, Izadnia, & Khan, 1999; Richter & Bradley, 1996; Mair, Schroder, Modalsi, & Maurer, 1974). Herbst (1996) reported that the globus sensation does not signify a psychological disorder, but rather a dysmotility of the upper esophageal or pharangeal muscles. Orenstein et al. (1999) reported that although originally considered to represent a psychogenic etiology, the globus sensation might have an organic basis. She delineates the differential diagnoses of dysphagia in children and adolescents as: (1) structural causes, (2) functional causes, (3) miscellaneous causes (including the globus sensation). Due to the large number of organic conditions that can cause the globus sensation, diagnostic errors exist with some documented rates as high as 25% (Guggenheim, 2000).

Gray (1983) postulated that minor pharyngeal irritation could initiate the globus sensation in which interprandial dry swallowing frequency increases as subjects try to "dislodge" the foreign body. Paradoxically this dry swallowing habit has been postulated as an indirect cause of the symptom with a subsequent increase in dry swallowing perpetrating a vicious cycle (Clouse et al., 1999).

Data from studies in adults are controversial as to whether GERD is the cause of the globus sensation. Whitehead and Schuster (1985) reported that from 50% to 90% of adult patients who present with a lump in their throat have reflux esophagitis or other peptic diseases causing pain in the throat. Moloy and Charter (1982) found that treatment of patients referred to an otolaryngology clinic for the globus symptom was unrelated to treatment response of reflux symptoms even with antireflux therapy. They reported no etiologic relationship between the globus symptom and GERD; rather, they stated that GERD and the globus sensation are independent phenomena that sometimes occur in the same individual.

Psychological Explanation

Psychological abnormalities are detected inconsistently in patients with globus, (Rasquin-Weber, Hyman, Cucchiara, Fleisher, & Hyams et al., 1999). Causal relationships between emotional abnormalities and globus have not been established, although patients with globus report a greater number of severe life events than controls over the year preceding symptom onset (Clouse, 1999).

The early psychoanalytic theorists described the globus sensation as "suppressed crying" occurring in times of strong emotion. Kanner was the first to describe the globus sensation as "globus hystericus," implying a diagnosis of conversion hysteria as the cause of the symptom. Data, however, suggest that the designation of hysteria is inappropriate since studies indicate that depressive, obsessive, and hypochondriachal symptoms are more characteristic of patients with the globus sensation than are histrionic features (Cook, Dent, & Collins, 1989; Lehtinen & Puhakka, 1976; Linder, 1973). Despite the lack of data for globus symptom as a psychological disorder, the etiology is still reported as "Psychological problems lead to the physical sensation of a lump in the throat that causes difficulty or discomfort in swallowing" (Finkenbine & Miele, 2004, p. 78).

The globus sensation exists in patients with significant psychiatric disease who do not have underlying esophageal disease. However, if other esophageal symptoms such as dysphagia or odynophagia are missed, globus may be wrongly attributed to emotional causes. This experience can lead to the erroneous assumption that since *some* patients present with globus in association with severe emotional symptoms, then the etiology for *all* patients who have globus is emotional.

Biopsychosocial Explanation

The biopsychosocial conceptualization of the etiology of the globus symptom recognizes the complicated and causal ways in which both organic and psychologic factors interact (Richter & Bradley, 1996). Yet the mechanisms for how these factors interact are unknown. In children and adolescents, these pathways are affected by the child's age, physical condition, temperament, and environmental factors, particularly the family. If a medical etiology for the globus sensation is determined, psychological and environmental factors can still contribute to the intensity of the symptom and to its maintenance. Likewise, if no physical findings have been diagnosed for the globus symptom, the physical sequelae of food refusal and constant throat clearing can affect physical functioning.

Richter and Bradley (1996) reported that both physiological and psychological stressors frequently trigger spastic esophageal disorders. They suggest that psychological factors may relate to the genesis of globus in four different domains: (1) stress may initiate globus, (2) patients with anxiety and depression may experience altered sensory mechanisms and the perception of discomfort, (3) psychophysiological reactions may include components that contribute to the globus sensation and the patient's reaction to it, and (4) psychological traits related to illness behavior may define the small subset of patients who will seek medical attention for this symptom.

Psychological disturbances are more common in patients who have globus sensation alone without obvious organic disease. Recent conceptualizations of panic disorders suggest that biologic and hypochondriacal traits predispose individuals to misinterpret and catastrophize body sensations, intensifying them. As with other individuals who are highly sensitive to their bodily cues, often known as "symptom reporters," globus can occur from normal physiological stimuli that are abnormally perceived (Pennebaker, 1982).

Globus has also been conceptualized as a symptom that is the result of conditioned learning responses. Williams and Hirsch (1988) suggest that the both the globus sensation and subsequent food refusal can reflect "learning" situations, which may be positively reinforced or negatively reinforced. For example, a child presenting with the globus symptom may receive additional attention and encouragement to eat (positive reinforcement). An adolescent may begin choking at a meal during which there is a family argument, which then stops with the sudden attention to the choking episode (negative reinforcement).

Chatoor et al. (1988) conceptualized the globus symptom and the subsequent food refusal in children as a posttraumatic stress response, which occurs after an experienced or observed traumatic choking episode. Parents and children distinctly remember the incident. Subsequently, the child becomes afraid to eat solid food and self-restricts out of fear, eating only soft foods or liquids. Other factors such as parental responses, existence of anxiety in the child or parent, and parental advice-seeking behavior contribute to the creation and maintenance of this sensation.

Diagnosis and Assessment

The criteria for diagnosis of globus sensation include positive identification of specific symptoms and the exclusion of structural and metabolic disorders, a pathology-based motor disorder, or pathological reflux (Clouse et al., 1999). Because of the chronicity of this symptom, organic etiologies need to be ruled out; however, extensive diagnostic testing must be carefully evaluated since it potentially can further increase anxiety about possible physical problems and thereby delay effective psychosocial treatment.

Deary, Wilson, Harris, and MacDougall, (1995) developed a 10-item throat questionnaire, the Glasgow-Edinburgh Throat Scale (GETS) to assess the severity of globus symptom in adults. The scale provides a quick quantitative estimate of throat symptoms for clinicians and it allows for following the progression of symptoms over time in response to different treatment modalities. There is no similar assessment tool for children or adolescents.

Once medical issues have been ruled out, the physician needs to clearly report diagnostic findings and then work toward reinforcing health-promoting behaviors in the child and the family (Drossman, 1998). Without a definitive reporting that the physical findings are normal, further exploration of psychological and environmental factors maybe resisted: the patients and his or her parents might still hold on to the belief that a physical cause for the symptom has yet to be found. Thus, during the diagnostic phase the physician has an opportunity to simultaneously validate the reality of the patient's physical complaint and to educate the patient and family to a biopsychosocial approach that physical, psychological, and environmental factors are not mutually exclusive.

Psychological Factors

Psychological factors to explore include:

- Does the patient exhibit anxiety symptoms?
- Does the child have a prior history of panic attacks?
- Has the child's or adolescent's mood changed?
- Have there been psychological ramifications of having this symptom? Has social anxiety increased? Is there school avoidance?

Environmental Factors

Environmental factors that should be assessed include:

- Is the globus symptom a reaction to a traumatic choking experience, either experienced or observed?
- Is the child receiving any secondary gain from this symptom, from the family or at school?
- Does the child have a supportive network of family or peers?
- Are the child's or adolescent's family able to set limits and to follow through with treatment guidelines?
- Does anyone else in the family have this symptom?

Treatment

There is neither theoretical consensus as to the etiology of the globus syndrome nor a single treatment of established efficacy (Bishop & Riley, 1988). Wilson (1992) suggests a common-sense approach to the treatment of globus: antiacid therapy (although the dyspepsia will respond more readily than the globus), relaxation exercises in tense, anxious individuals, and antidepressant therapy in the clinically depressed. Evidence-based results of treatment modalities for the globus sensation in the pediatric and adolescent population are lacking: treatment data come from case studies.

Culbert et al. (1996) reported the successful treatment of 5 children with dysphagia and food aversion in a series of 5 case studies. The treatment strategies used included: educational interventions, self-hypnosis, and cognitive behavioral suggestions. The educational component consisted of information regarding normal swallowing and identifying the connections between the child's thoughts about eating and his or her physiological responses. The self-hypnosis component included: relaxation techniques, mental imagery that allows the child to individualize body-mind linkages, *in vitro* rehearsal, desensitization to eating situations, and posthypnotic suggestions that link positive feelings and comfort to meals and swallowing. Cognitive-behavioral strategies focused on identifying negative self-talk cycles around feeding and swallowing and learning positive self-talk strategies.

Chatoor et al. (1988) conceptualized the globus sensation and food refusal after either experiencing or observing a serious choking incident as a posttraumatic stress disorder in children. Their treatment focused on two principal goals: to get the child to eat and to decrease the parental/caregiver anxiety about separation issues, which they believed is the underlying dynamic maintaining the symptom. Food refusal was treated by a food desensitization program, which included progressive relaxation to deal with anticipatory anxiety over choking, a food hierarchy from most to least feared food, and an *in vitro* desensitization procedure culminating in an *in vivo* desensitization experience. Concurrent family therapy was provided to ensure that parental anxiety was not a contributory factor to the maintenance of the symptom.

Results indicated that food consumption increased for each of the children following treatment.

Donahue, Thevenin and Runyon (1997) reported the successful treatment case study of a 12-year-old girl presenting with globus and weight loss. Treatment modalities included detailed behavioral assessment of negative and positive consequences of the symptom. A food hierarchy was established. "Training meals" used specific throat relaxation techniques and positive mental imagery prior to actually trying the next food on the hierarchy. A list of reinforcers was established and used for achievement of goals. Oberfeld (1981) reported the successful treatment of an adolescent girl with globus and weight loss using family therapy.

As with other pediatric functional disorders, anecdotal data indicate that until the patient and family are convinced that physical etiologies have been ruled out, behavioral/psychological treatment will not proceed smoothly (Drossman, 1998; Wolff, 1973). Validation that the symptom is real is important in obtaining the trust of the patient and the family. A review of physical testing results with the patient and family is important to facilitate a cognitive shift from focus on physical issues to focus on effective psychological or behavioral treatment.

Dubowitz and Hersov (1976) recommend that the objectives of psychological intervention in children and adolescents with the globus sensation include: (1) a specific behavioral plan to decrease the effect of the globus sensation with respect to fear of swallowing and food refusal, (2) improvement of the patient's functioning by eliminating any "sick role" behavior, and (3) alteration of parental perceptions from having a sick child to a potential healthy and normally developing one. Figure 4.2 is an algorithm for the treatment of the globus sensation.

New Directions

Globus is a symptom easy to identify clinically, with a complicated etiology. Physical, psychological, and environmental factors co-occur in a variety of combinations or sequences. Future issues to be explored with respect to the globus symptom in children and adolescents include:

1. Clarification of the definition of the globus symptom: What are the subgroups of this symptom? Does it include problems with swallowing? Is it a posttraumatic event?
2. Epidemiological data of the globus sensation in children and adolescents needs to be obtained.
3. An adaptation of the GETS for children and adolescents as an adjunctive diagnostic tool is needed.
4. An assessment of the impact of this symptom on the quality of life for children and adolescents should be assessed: How much does the globus symptom interfere with the child's participation in age-appropriate activities?

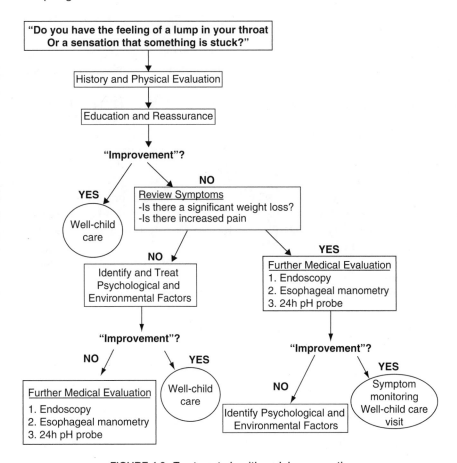

FIGURE 4.2. Treatment algorithm globus sensation

5. Evidence-based research in dealing with this problem is important to determine what works best for children and adolescents presenting with this symptom. When is psychopharmacological intervention warranted and is it effective? Is progressive relaxation helpful in maintaining improvement after behavioral treatment?

Proposed Biopsychosocial Treatment Plan for Globus Sensation

Treatment of this symptom is difficult because of unclear etiologies, its recurrence, and its chronicity, leading some to suggest that it is a symptom to be managed rather than treated. Following is an outline of the measures to take in each session of treatment.

Session 1: Team Building and History Taking

a. Reassure the child or adolescent and the parents that the globus symptom improves in time and that a team of professionals is coordinating the care.
b. Reassurance by the physician that there is nothing "stuck," and review of medical procedures which have already been performed and the results.
c. Obtain a detailed description of the problem, a history of its course, and if the child has either experienced or observed a severe choking episode.
d. Obtain a detailed history of the child's medical problems, developmental history, and current level of functioning at home, at school, and with peers. Determine if the child's symptom is serving a functional role in the family system.
e. Evaluate the psychological functioning of the child. Symptoms of mood disorder, phobic avoidance, or panic anxiety should be explored in the interview and with the use of normed questionnaires.

   1. The child or adolescent should complete the March Anxiety Scale for Children (MASC) (March, Parker, Sullivan, Stallings, and Conners, 1997) and Childhood Depression Inventory (CDI) (Kovacs, 1985).
   2. The caregiver should complete the Child Behavior Check List (CBCL) (Achenbach, 1999).

Session 2: Education

a. Educate the patient and family regarding the normal functioning of the esophagus, using books, pictures, and diagrams. Provide information regarding the relationship between psychological and physical factors.
b. If a medical problem has been identified, reinforce compliance with the treatment plan and coordinate care with the physician.
c. If an anxiety disorder or an affective disorder has been identified, make sure that the child or adolescent is treated for this.
d. Discuss how cognitive-behavioral treatments are helpful in altering the cognitive-physiologic feedback loop.

Sessions 3–8. Cognitive Behavioral Management

a. Teach techniques including: progressive muscle relaxation and visual imagery of the movement of the food through the esophagus. Learn cognitive-behavioral strategies to develop increased awareness of negative self-talk around feeding and swallowing such as "The food is going to get stuck" during eating. Learn positive self-talk strategies and rehearse alternative statements.

b. Construct hierarchy of food consistency from least to most difficult foods to swallow. Use a practice *in vitro* rehearsal using a standard systematic desensitization (or guided exposure) paradigm, as increasingly higher levels of the food hierarchy are introduced. The relaxation procedure is to be performed before and after eating.

c. Posthypnotic suggestions to link positive feelings/association of confidence and comfort to meals and swallowing.

d. Establish with patient specific goals to be met for each session and provide mutually agreed upon rewards/reinforcers.

e. Have practice training meals to ensure that the patient is correctly using behavioral tools and imagery.

f. Review environmental factors such as parental anxiety and concern that may be providing secondary gain to the patient

If treatment is not effective despite compliance with the treatment regimen, medical issues should be reevaluated.

Gastroesophageal Reflux

Gastroesophageal reflux (GER) is a frequent phenomenon of the involuntary passage of gastric contents into the esophagus (Orenstein, 1999) in infants and children. GER can consist of gas (burp) or fluid (wet burp, "spitting up" in infants). In most children and adults, this is a normal process that occurs several to many times a day, without fluid coming back to the mouth (Blanchard, 2005; Vandenplas & Hassall, 2002). This process serves to relieve gastric distension. Parents of infants actively promote this process by burping their infants directly after feeding.

Although reflux is a normal physiological response that occurs at all ages, many pediatric gastroenterologists report a continuum ranging from physiological GER and leading to GERD, a condition in which severe symptoms and complications occur secondarily to the refluxate (Jones, 2001; Orenstein et al., 1999; Vandenplas & Hassall, 2002).

Definition of Condition

GER is a prevalent gastrointestinal problem in children: many infants have recurrent problems of spitting up and vomiting during the first year of life. The gastric contents can vary and includes saliva, ingested foods and drinks, and gastric, pancreatic, or biliary secretions (Vandenplas, 2000). Most episodes of reflux are into the distal esophagus, brief and asymptomatic. However, GER can range from the occasional "burp and spit-up" to life-threatening malnutrition from severe regurgitation with failure to thrive.

Regurgitation is the passage of refluxed gastric contents into the oral pharynx (Vandenplas, 2000). The term regurgitation is used if the reflux dribbles effortlessly into or out of the mouth and is restricted to infancy (from birth to 12 months) (Vandenplas & Hegar, 2000). Regurgitation by the baby with GER is conceptualized as a pressure release phenomenon (Orenstein, 1997).

Vomiting, a synonym for emesis, occurs when the refluxed material comes out of the mouth "with a certain degree of strength" or "more or less vigorously," usually involuntarily and with the sensation of nausea (Vandenplas & Hegar, 2000). Vomiting is described as the tip of the iceberg in relation to the incidence of GER episodes (Vandenplas, 2000).

Epidemiology

GER varies largely according to age, usually beginning at 2 to 3 months of age. GER is extremely common in infancy, with approximately half of all infants up to 3 months, and two thirds of infants between 4 and 6 months of age having symptoms of regurgitation, which occur daily in almost 70% of 4-month-old infants. The vast majority of these infants have effortless regurgitation with no apparent GER-associated complications and spontaneous resolution of their symptoms by 9 to 12 months of age (Lee & Rudolph, 2001). The peak age for reporting 4 or more episodes of regurgitation was at 5 months of age (23%), which decreased to 7% at 7 months. Daily regurgitation is present in only 5% of infants at 1 year of age (Salvatore & Vandenplas, 2003). There is no difference in the incidence of regurgitation between breastfed and formula-fed infants (Orenstein, Izadnia & Khan, 1999; Vandenplas, 2000).

Course and Prognosis

Regurgitation is common in infants and typically has a spontaneous resolution (Salvatore & Vandenplas, 2003). In most cases regurgitation resolves by 12 to 18 months of age (Kumar & Sarvanthanan, 2003). If GER persists beyond 4 years of age, there is less than a 50% chance of spontaneous resolution (Zeiter & Hyams, 1999).

Etiology

Transient relaxation of the lower esophageal sphincter (TRLES) appears to be the most common mechanism leading to GER. During TRLES, both the LES and the crural diaphragm are inhibited for between 10-60 seconds, and this inhibition is mediated by a brainstem reflex (Zeiter & Hyams, 1999). Other mechanisms involved in GER include: (1) increased intra-abdominal pressure, (2) reduced esophageal capacitance, (3) decreased gastric compliance, and (4) delayed gastric emptying.

Esophageal capacitance contributes to the frequency of GER in infants due to: (1) a shorter esophagus, (2) smaller capacity of the esophagus, (3) a recumbent posture and therefore the lack of gravity. These factors make it more likely that the refluxed material in the infant will fill the esophagus and pass to the pharynx (Figure 4.3).

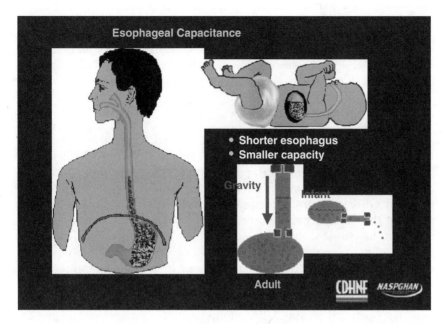

FIGURE 4.3. Esophageal capacitance (Reproduced by permission of CDHNF/ NASPGHAN from the CME CD-ROM *Pediatric Gastroesophageal Reflux Disease, Evaluation and Management*, developed by the Children's Digestive Health and Nutrition Foundation and the North American Society for Pediatric Gastroenterology, Hepatology and Nutrition.)

There appear to be genetic influences on the prevalence of GER. The concordance rate for GER is higher in monozygotic than in dyzygotic twins. There is also an increase in GER symptoms seen in relatives of patients with GERD (Salvatore & Vandenplas, 2003).

Clinical Presentation

The usual manifestations of GER are vomiting, regurgitation, and nausea. Uncommon symptoms can include: dysphagia, failure to thrive (FTT), noncardiac chest pain, heartburn, anemia, recurrent pneumonia, apnea, and general irritability in infants (Faubion & Zein, 1998). Orenstein (1997) differentiates between the regurgitant reflux in infants and adults, citing that infants do not have the social pressures that adults do to keep supraesophageal reflux from exiting the mouth: she states, "regurgitatant reflux occurs nearly exclusively in young infants in part because of their uncivilized nature" (p. 115S).

Although GER is a commonly occurring symptom in infants, it can be a source of severe worry for parents, who become extremely anxious with the infant. Complicated interactions around feeding can develop, and they are potentially very difficult for first-time parents or anxious parents.

Diagnosis and Assessment

The North American Society of Pediatric Gastroenterology and Nutrition (Rudolph et al., 2001) states that in most cases a history and physical exam are sufficient to reliably diagnose GER and to initiate management.

Medical Treatment

Infants with typical symptoms of uncomplicated GER should be treated without investigation or other procedures. NASPGN (2001) reports that in the infant with uncomplicated GER, parental education, reassurance, and anticipatory guidance are recommended. Physicians should reassure concerned parents that GER is a normal phenomenon in infants, recognized as "spitting up," and that this phenomenon occurs universally. Giving parents practical advice on how to feed the infant and an actual demonstration of antireflux techniques have been shown to be helpful (Vandenplas, 2000). Studies have documented the effects of parental reassurance by placebo-controlled studies, which showed similar efficacies between the placebo and reassurance.

Thickening of infant formula and a short trial of hypoallergenic formula are other treatment options. If symptoms worsen or do not improve by 12 to 18 months, reevaluation for complications of GER is recommended. Diseases caused by GER can be investigated specifically and managed with accurately defined therapy. However, for children who suffer intractable GER with secondary complications, failure of therapy could mean surgical intervention (Jones, 2001).

Psychosocial Treatment

A child with GER can affect the whole family. Parents have concerns regarding their ability to successfully parent; they worry about the health of their child and the disruption of other family relationships. Often the first-year feeding experiences are negative. Keeping a feeding and behavioral diary to monitor symptoms and to document signs of improvement provides objective information and is helpful to alleviate fear and decrease anxiety.

If parents are particularly anxious, or if they have had a difficult pregnancy or fertility issues, extra reassurance is warranted. Anticipatory guidance by the pediatrician can be a preventive step in decreasing the possibility of a vulnerable child syndrome where parental anxiety about the child can have a future impact on the child's psychosocial development.

Gastroesophageal Reflux Disease

Vandenplas and Hassall (2002) and Mason (2000) describe gastroesophageal reflux disease (GERD) as "a spectrum of disease that can best be defined as the symptoms and/or signs of esophageal or adjacent organ injury secondary to the reflux of gastric contents into the esophagus or, beyond, into the oral cavity or airways" (p. 120). GERD results from an increased frequency or duration of reflux episodes during which the increased noxiousness of the refluxate can cause dangerous consequences secondarily to GER (Sunku, Marino, & Sockolow, 2000). GERD is also defined as abnormal reflux or GER with identified complications, which are associated with mucosal damage or symptoms severe enough to impair quality of life (Salvatore & Vandenplas, 2003).

Epidemiology

Five percent to 9% of infants have troublesome GERD. In older children, the prevalence of GERD is still undefined, but seems more resistant to complete resolution. Determination of the exact prevalence of GERD at any age is difficult because of self-treatment or lack of medical referral (Salvatore & Vandenplas, 2003). GERD is the third top discharge diagnosis for children: 64,814 (3.5%) of all discharges of hospitalized children had GERD-related disorders (Blanchard, 2005).

Course and Prognosis

In older children, GERD has a less benign prognosis and more frequently requires medical help. Because treatment for GERD has become common, it is impossible to document the natural course of the illness. High-risk groups, including children with cystic fibrosis (CF), neurological impairment, and esophagyeal atresia, are more likely to have persistent disease. Whether the treatment of regurgitation in young infants changes the incidence or severity of symptoms is unknown. Neurological patients are likely to have the most severe reflux disease and the poorest response to treatment. Reflux is likely to get worse with age (Salvatore & Vandenplas, 2003).

Unusual complications of GERD include esophagitis, anemia, respiratory problems, such as cough, apnea, and recurrent wheezing, and failure to thrive (Kumar & Saravanthanan, 2003). The lack of long-term reports, the complexity of pathophysiology involving environmental and genetic factors, and the absence of pathognomic symptoms for the disease itself or its complications make it difficult to predict which child will continue to have GERD into and during adult life with the resulting risks for severe complications (Salvatore & Vandenplas, 2003).

Etiology

Premature infants and children with severe neurodevelopmental problems or congenital esophageal anomalies are particularly at risk (Kumar & Sarvananthan, 2003). The majority of children with severe neurological impairment are diagnosed with GERD. The neurological disease itself may cause delayed esophageal clearance and delayed gastric emptying; most of these children are bedridden (gravity improves esophageal clearance) and many are constipated, which increases abdominal pressure (Vandenplas & Hegar, 2000).

Experimental findings suggest that in adults the relationship between stress and increased refluxed symptoms may be due to the subgroup of patients characterized by high levels of anxiety: anxious patients may devote excessive attention to a wide variety of esophageal events and label them as painful. There is also evidence that when chronically anxious patients with GERD are exposed to prolonged stress, somatavisceral information from the esophagus is affected: low intensity esophageal events are perceived as reflux symptoms (Richter & Bradley, 1996). Thus for a subgroup of patients with GERD stress can lead to typical symptoms of heartburn, but without a physiological increase in acid reflux. Thus, there is an abnormal perception of normal physiological function, rather than a normal perception of abnormal physiological processes (Drossman, 1998).

Clinical Presentation

Typical GI symptoms for GERD include frequent emesis, burping, gagging, failure to thrive, chest or abdominal pain, or dysphagia. In the pediatric age group, GERD remains the most common organic cause of esophagus-related pain (Kumar & Saranathan, 2003).

The severity of symptoms from GERD can vary from intermittent burping to persistent emesis. Children with GERD, however, do not always present with typical symptoms; they can present with extraesophageal manifestations including: hoarseness, frequent coughing, asthma, and recurrent pneumonia (Carr et al., 2000).

In neurologically disabled children, regurgitation is the most common symptom of reflux; however, complications are frequent, including recurrent pulmonary disease, anemia, and weight loss. Food avoidance and behavioral changes can also be subtle symptoms of GERD in this group (Faubion & Zein, 1998).

Diagnosis and Assessment

A complete history and physical exam are the first steps in the diagnosis of GERD. Further assessment of GERD and the diagnostic therapeutic approaches vary according to age, clinical presentation, and procedure facilities. An upper GI exam is useful for the evaluation of the presence of anatomic abnormalities, such as pyloric stenosis, malrotation, and annular pancreas in the vomiting infant as well as hiatal hernia and esophageal stricture in the older child (NASPGN, 2001). Long-term esophageal pH monitoring is recommended for the diagnosis of the patient suspected of unusual or atypical presentations of GERD (Vandenplas & Hegar, 2000). In the case of rapid relapse, severe symptoms, or suspected esophagitis, an endoscopy is recommended (NASPGN, 2001).

For the older child or adolescent with GERD, there is a potential for impact on functioning in age-appropriate arenas such as school, social activities, and participation in athletics. Our experience is that for the child/adolescent with GERD, functioning is most significantly affected by the following factors: (1) severity of symptoms, (2) the child/adolescent's self-conscious or level of anxiety about his or her symptoms, and (3) the family or caregiver reaction to symptoms. Thus from a biopsychosocial perspective, it is important to identify child/adolescent–related factors such as anxiety and environmental factors or school or family issues that may be contributing to stress or providing secondary gain for symptoms. These reactions to symptoms may be maintaining unnecessary illness-related behaviors such as school avoidance.

Recently, the Pediatric GERD Caregiver Impact Questionnaire in English and Spanish (PGCIQ) was developed to elucidate the impact of caring for a child with GERD. It is the first questionnaire which recognizes the biopsychosocial impact of this disorder by documenting the multidimensional impact of caring for an infant or young child with GERD (Kim, Keininger, Becker, & Crawley, 2005).

Treatment

Rudolph et al. (2001) recommend that in infants and toddlers with chronic vomiting or regurgitation and recurrent episodes of cough and wheezing, or in children/adolescents with coexisting symptoms of asthma and esophagitis, a 3-month trial of vigorous acid suppressant therapy be tried. For the treatment of heartburn in children or adolescents, lifestyle changes can be accompanied by 2- to 4-week therapeutic trial of a histamine 2 receptor antagonist (H2RA) or proton pump inhibitor (PPI). If symptoms persist or recur, the child can be referred for upper endoscopy with biopsy and in some cases long-term therapy. Rudolph et al. (2001) recommend that children and adolescents with GERD avoid caffeine, chocolate, and spicy foods that may provoke symptoms.

Kumar and Saranathan (2003) reviewed the results of evidence-based treatments for GERD in children. Their review from randomized controlled trials (RCT) found (1) 2 studies in infants and children under 2 years of age found that sodium alginate reduced the frequency of regurgitation at 8 to 14 days compared with a placebo, (2) domeperidone, feed thickeners, H2 antagonists, metoclopramide, proton pump inhibitors, and surgery were of unknown effectiveness (Cisapride has been withdrawn or restricted in several countries because of an association with heart rhythm abnormalities), and (3) positioning (either left lateral or prone) was not shown to be effective and data indicated that both prone and left lateral positions may be associated with higher risk of sudden infant death syndrome compared to supine positioning.

Surgery is considered for children who have persistent GERD or who cannot be weaned from their medical therapy. The Nissen fundoplication is the most common procedure. Recently laparoscopic procedures have been reported. However, while data indicate favorable outcomes, these data are based on case studies and have methodological problems with respect to subject selection (Rudolph et al., 2001.)

Richter and Bradley (1996) report data in adults that progressive muscle relaxation training can be a useful adjunct to traditional antireflux therapy in patients with GERD who also present with anxiety. Data showing the efficacy of relaxation techniques for children and adolescents with GERD are not available. The first author's anecdotal clinical experience indicates that for children with GERD who also have anxiety problems, relaxation techniques are helpful. They can serve as an adjunctive therapy for the child or adolescent as part of a "tool box" of strategies to help manage "worrying," which can also decrease the amount of discomfort that the child/adolescent experiences. If family factors have been identified that contribute to maintaining a "sick role," these need to be addressed so that functioning can continue at an age-appropriate level.

Prior to the first treatment session, obtain medical information from the pediatric gastroenterologist or pediatrician treating the child. The following outline includes the steps in the various treatment sessions for patients with GERD.

Session 1: Team Building and History Taking

a. Provide reassurance to the child and family that a team of professionals is coordinating care.
b. Obtain a detailed description of the course of the child's illness, developmental history, and current level of functioning at home, at school, and with peers.
c. Emphasize that *there is* a medical problem, *but* psychological factors may impact how the patient responds to the physical symptom: Are they sensitive to visceral discomfort and do they "worry" that their "pain/discomfort" is symptomatic of a life-threatening illness?
d. Have parents complete the CBCL (Achenbach, 1991).

Session 2: Evaluation of the Child and Education

a. Determine functioning at home and at school. Identify stressors for the child such as peer relationships, academic pressures, and family life. Are any activities being disrupted due to having GERD? Is the child or adolescent going to school on a regular basis?
b. Evaluate the psychological functioning of the child with particular attention to issues of anxiety. Have the child complete the MASC (March et al., 1997). Provide treatment if an anxiety disorder is diagnosed.
c. Provide information regarding a biopsychosocial conceptualization of GERD specific to the child or adolescent and discuss how cognitive-behavioral treatments are helpful in altering the cognitive-physiologic feedback loop.
d. Reinforce compliance with the medical treatment plan.

Sessions 3–6: Cognitive-Behavioral Management

a. Determine what actions can be taken with respect to management of stresses. Set specific goals for each session.

b. Teach techniques such as progressive relaxation and visualization to aid in relaxation.

c. Review issues such as parental anxiety or extra attention from classmates that may be contributing to the maintenance of behaviors secondary to a diagnosis of GERD.

New Directions

Pediatricians need to assess the impact of repetitive regurgitation on the health-related quality of life (HRQOL) of the patient and his or her family. Research is needed to define how and why pediatric patients may progress to persisting symptoms and complications and if a different GERD phenotype is related to genetic heterogeneity (Salvatore & Vandenplas, 2003).

Additional studies in children and adolescents are needed to determine whether and which adjunctive treatments such as hypnosis and progressive relaxation are effective in reducing either the frequency of symptoms or the patient's reporting of the intensity of the symptoms.

Esophageal Motility Disorders

Esophageal motility disorders are produced by a variety of abnormalities in the coordinated neuromuscular components responsible for esophageal peristalsis (Richter & Bradley, 1996). The primary symptoms are dysphagia and chest pain. Esophageal motility disorders occasionally produce distressing, life-threatening complications; but the symptoms are usually subtle and intermittent. Expanded diagnostic technology has facilitated the diagnosis of esophageal motility disorders in the body of the esophagus as well as the upper and lower esophageal sphincters.

Achalasia

Achalasia is an uncommon motility disorder characterized by failure of the LES and a lack of propulsive peristalsis in the esophageal body. Symptoms include difficulty in swallowing, regurgitation of food, cough due to overflow of fluids into the trachea, failure to gain weight, and chest pain. Patients eat slowly and often drink large amounts of fluids with meals. The incidence of achalasia has been estimated as 1 in 10,000; fewer than 5% of those patients with symptoms are younger than 15 years of age. It is uncommon under 5 years of age. The diagnosis is typically confirmed with an esophageal manometry. Treatment for achalasia can include pharmacotherapy, pneumatic dilation, and Heller's operation (myotomy), a procedure that splits the LES, which now can be performed laparoscopically (Herbst, 1996).

Diffuse Esophageal Spasm

Diffuse esophageal spasm (DES) is characterized by variable manometric patterns and symptoms. Patients have motor abnormalities that fluctuate between normal and abnormal. Symptoms include: intermittent chest pain or dysphagia that is usually nonprogressive. Esophageal manometry usually defines the motor abnormalities in the distal esophagus and is the most useful test. Treatment modalities are limited, nonspecific measures include avoiding extremely hot or cold food and eating in an upright position in a relaxed atmosphere (Herbst, 1996).

Although psychophysiological factors have been shown to effect esophageal functioning, the pathophysiology of spastic esophageal motility disorders is poorly understood. Environmental stresses such as stressful interviews or noxious noise have been shown to contribute to abnormal esophageal contractions. Stress may also increase LES pressure as well as contractions in the esophageal body (Richter & Bradley, 1996). Several studies in adults have demonstrated that esophageal disorders are associated with high level of psychological distress as a result of elevated scores on self-report measures of psychological distress, most commonly depression, anxiety disorder, and somatization disorder (Clouse & Lustman, 1988). In adults, treatment of spastic esophageal motility disorders includes psychopharmacotherapy. The data from a double-blind study in adults show that low-dose therapy with trazadone improved symptoms (Clouse, Lustman, Eckert, Ferney, & Griffith, 1987).

An essential treatment component for children and their patients is confident reassurance that the patient's pain is due to an esophageal motility disorder rather than cardiac disease or some other life-threatening problem. Reassurance decreases the child's anxiety and facilitates the acceptance of the diagnosis and the treatment regimen.

Nonspecific Esophageal Motility Disorders in Children without GER

The classification of nonspecific esophageal motility disorders (NEMDs) has been used to describe manometry findings that are abnormal but not diagnostic of an established motility disorder such as achalasia or DES. In a study of 154 children with upper GI symptoms, 13 or 8% were diagnosed with NEMDs. The variable clinical course suggests that NEMDs in the pediatric age group represents an evolving group of motility disorders. Children with NEMDs exhibit a diverse array of symptoms including: vomiting, dysphagia, chest pain, food impaction, and epigastric pain. Data from this study group of patients aged 4 to 18 years indicated that NEMDs represent a common group of esophageal abnormalities in children with upper gastrointestinal tract symptoms without GER. Food impaction appears to be a relatively frequent complication, and NEMDs should be considered in children who have this finding (Rosario et al., 1999).

No single therapeutic approach has been found to relieve symptoms, and no correlation was found between therapeutic intervention and the clinical course of the 13 patients identified with NEMDs.

New Directions

Data on the epidemiology of the functional esophageal disorders such as globus sensation in children and adolescents needs to be obtained. Explanations of the fundamental mechanisms of symptom occurrence from a biopsychosocial perspective need to be clarified. Studies that evaluate the efficiency of different treatment approaches with each of the esophageal disorders with respect to outcome are needed. Further prospective research is needed to determine how esophageal disorders impact the child's development in unique ways, and if so, what the psychological and social sequelae are for both the child and the family.

REFERENCES

Achenbach, T. (1991). *Manual of the Child Behavior Checklist* (CBCL). Burlington, VT: University Associates of Psychiatry.

Bishop, L. C., & Riley, W. T. (1988). The psychiatric management of the globus syndrome. *General Hospital Psychiatry, 9*, 214–219.

Bithoney, W. G., & Dubowitz, H. (1985). Organic concomitants of nonorganic failure to thrive. In D. Drotar (Ed.), *New directions in failure to thrive: Implications for research and practice* (pp. 47–68). New York: Plenum.

Blanchard, S. (2005). Diagnosis and treatment of gastroesophageal reflux. Patient care conference presentation. Rainbow Babies & Children's Hospital, Cleveland, OH.

Bradley, P. J., & Narula, A. (1987). Clinical aspects of pseudodysphagia. *Journal of Laryngology and Otology, 101*, 689–694.

Carr, M., Nguyen, A., Nagy, M., Poje, C., Pizzuto, M., & Brodsky, L. (2000). Clinical presentation as a guide to the identification of GERD in children. *International Journal of Pediatric Otorhinolaryngology, 54*, 27–32.

Chatoor, I., Conley, C., & Dickson, L. (1988). Food refusal after an incident of choking: A post-traumatic eating disorder. *Journal of the American Academy of Child and Adolescent Psychiatry, 27*, 105–110.

Clouse, R. E., & Lustman, P. J. (1988). Psychiatric illness and contraction abnormalities of the oesphagus. *New England Journal of Medicine, 309*, 1337–1342.

Clouse, R. E., Lustman, P. J., Eckert, T. C., Ferney, D. M., Griffith L. S. (1987). Low-dose trazodone for symptomatic patients with esophageal contraction abnormalities. A double-blind, placebo-controlled trial. *Gastroenterology, 92*(4), 1027–1036.

Clouse, R. E., Richter, J. E., Heading, R. C., Janseens, J., & Wilson, J. A. (1999). Functional esophageal disorders. *Gut, 45*(Suppl. 2), II31.

Cook, I. J., Dent, J., & Collins, S. M. (1989). Upper esophageal sphincter tone and reactivity to stress in patients with a history of globus sensation. *Digestive Diseases and Sciences, 34*, 672.

Culbert, T. P., Kajander, R. L., Kohen, D. P., & Reaney, J. B. (1996, October). Hypnobehavioral approaches for school-age children with dysphagia and food aversion: a case series. *Journal of Developmental and Behavioral Pediatrics, 17*(5), 335–341.

Deary, I. J., Wilson, J. A., Harris, M. B., & MacDougall, G. (1995, February). Globus pharyngis: Development of a symptom assessment scale. *Journal of Psychosomatic Research, 39*(2), 203–213.

Deary, I. J., Wilson, J. A., & Kelly, S. W. (1995, November–December). Globus pharyngis, personality, and psychological distress in the general population. *Psychosomatics, 36*(6), 570–577.

Donahue, B., Thevenin D. M., & Runyon, M. K. (1997). Behavioral treatment of conversion disorder in adolescence. A case example of globus hystericus. *Behavior Modification, 21*, 231–251.

Dubowitz, V., & Hersov, L. (1976). Management of children with non-organic (hysterical) disorders of motor function. *Developmental Medicine and Child Neurology, 18*, 358–368.

Farkkila, M. A., Ertama, L., Katila, H., Kuusi, K., Paavolainen, M., & Varis, K. (1994). Globus pharyngis, commonly associated with esophagael motility disorders. *American Journal of Gastroenterology, 89*(4), 503–508.

Faubion, W., & Zein, N. (1998). Gastroesophageal reflux in infants and children. *Mayo Clinic Proceedings, 73*, 166–173.

Finkenbine, R., & Miele, V. J. (2004). Globus hystericus: A brief review. *General Hospital Psychiatry, 26*, 78–82.

Gray, J. P. (1983). The relationship of the inferior constrictor swallow and globus hystericus or the hypopharyngeal syndrome. *Journal of Laryngology Otology, 97*, 607–618.

Guggenheim, F. G. (2000). Somatoform disorders. In H. I. Kaplan & V. A. Sadock (Eds.), *Comprehensive textbook of psychiatry* (7th ed., pp. 1504–1532). Baltimore: Lippincott Williams and Wilkins.

Herbst, J. J. (1996). Achalasia and other motor disorders. In R. Wylie and J. S. Hyams (Eds.), *Pediatric gastrointestinal disease pathophysiology diagnosis management* (pp. 391–402). Philadelphia: Saunders.

Jones, A. B. (2001, October). Gastroesophageal reflux in infants and children. When to reassure and when to go further. *Canadian Family Physician, 47*, 2045–50, 2053.

Kim, J, Keininger, D. L., Becker, S., & Crawley, J. A. (2005). Simultaneous development of the Pediatric GERD Caregiver Impact Questionnaire (PGCIQ) in American English and Spanish. *Health Quality of Life Outcomes. 3*(1), 5.

Kovacs, M. (1985). The Childrens Depression Inventory (CDI). *Psychopharmacology Bulletin, 21*(4), 995–998.

Kumar, Y., & Sarvananthan, R. (2003). Gastro-esophageal reflux in children. *Clinical Evidence, 10*, 397–405.

Lee, P., & Rudolph, C. (2001). Gastroesophageal reflux in infants and children. *Advances in Pediatrics, 48*, 301–329.

Lehtinen, V., & Puhakka, H. (1976, January). A psychosomatic approach to the globus hystericus syndrome. *Acta Psychiatrica Scandinavica, 53*(1), 21–28.

Liebowitz, M. R. (1987). Globus hystericus and panic attacks (letter). *American Journal of Psychiatry, 143*, 917–918.

Linder, A. E. (1973). Emotional factors in gastrointestinal illness. *Roche Medical Monograph Series International Congress no. 304*. Excerpta Medica. New York: American Elsevier.

Mair, I., W. S., Schroder, K. E., Modalsi, B., Maurer, H. J. (1974). Aetiological aspects of globus symptom. *Journal of Laryngology and Otology, 88*, 1033–1040.

March, J. S., Parker, J. D., Sullivan, K., Stallings, P., & Conners, C. K. (1997). Multidimensional Anxiety Scale for Children (MASC): Factor structure, reliability, and validity. *Journal of the American Academy of Child and Adolescent Psychiatry, 36*(12), 1645–1646.

Mason, D. B. (2000). Gastroesophageal reflux in children: A guide for the advanced practice nurse. *Nursing Clinics of North America, 35*(1), 15–36.

Mitrany, E. (1992). Atypical eating disorders. *Journal of Adolescent Health, 13*, 400–402.

Moloy, P. J., & Charter, R. (1982). The globus syndrome. *Archives of Otolaryngology, 108*, 740–744.

Moser, G., Wenzel-Abatzi, T. A., Stelzeneder, M., Wenzel, T., Weber, U., Wiesnagrotzki, S. et al. (1998, June 22). Globus sensation: Pharyngoesphageal function, psychometric and psychological findings, and follow-up in 88 patients. *Archives of Internal Medicine, 158*(12), 1365–1373.

Oberfield, R. A. (1981). Family therapy with adolescents: Treatment of a teenage girl with globus hystericus and weight loss. *Journal of American Academy of Child Psychiatry, 20*, 822–833.

Orenstein, S. (1994). Gastroesophageal reflux. In P. E. Hyman (Ed.), *Pediatric gastrointestinal motility disorders* (pp. 55–88). New York: Academy Professional Information Services.

Orenstein, S. R. (1997). Infantile reflux: Different from adult reflux. *American Journal of Medicine, 104*, 114S–119S.

Orenstein, S. R. (1999). Gastroesophageal reflux. *Pediatrics in Review, 20*(1); 24–80.

Orenstein, S. R., Izadnia, F., & Khan, S. (1999). Gastroesophageal reflux disease in children. In G. E. Katz (Ed.), *Gasteroenterology Clinics of North America* (pp. 947–969). Philadelphia: W. B. Saunders.

Pehlivanturk, B., & Unal, F. (2002). Conversion disorder in children and adolescents: A 4-year follow-up study. *Journal of Psychosomatic Research, 52*, 187–191.

Pennebaker, J. W. (1982). *The psychology of physical symptoms.* New York: Springer.

Rasquin-Weber, A., Hyman, P. E., Cucchiara, S., Fleisher, D. R., Hyams, J. S., Milla, P. J., & Staiano, A. (1999). Childhood functional gastrointestinal disorders. *Gut 45* (Suppl. 11): 1160–1168.

Ravich, W. J., Wilson, R. S., Jones, B., & Donner, M. W. (1989). Psychogenic dysphagia and globus: Reevaluation of 23 patients. *Dysphagia, 4*(1), 35–38. (Erratum in [1990] *Dysphagia, 4*(4), 244).

Richter, J. E., & Bradley, L. C. (1996, October). Psychophysiological interactions in esophageal diseases. *Seminars in Gastrointestinal Disease, 7*(4), 169–184.

Rosario, J. A., Medow, M. S., Halata, M. S., Bostwick, H. E., Newman, L. J., & Schwarz, S. M. (1999). Berezin. Nonspecific esophageal motility disorders in children without gastroesophageal reflux. *Journal of Pediatric Gastroenterology and Nutrition, 28*(5), 480–485.

Rudolph, C. D., Mazur, L. J., Liptak, G. S., Baker, R. D., Boyle, J. T., Colletti, R. B. et al. (2001). North American Society for Pediatric Gastroenterology and Nutrition. Guidelines for evaluation and treatment of gastroesophageal reflux in infants and children: recommendations of the North American Society for Pediatric Gastroenterology and Nutrition. *Journal of Pediatric Gastroenterology and Nutrition, 32*(Suppl. 2), S1–S31.

Salvatore, S., & Vandenplas, Y. (2003). Gastro-esophageal reflux disease and motility disorders. *Best Practice and Research Clinical Gastroenetrology, 17*(2), 163–179.

Shiomi, Y., Shiomi, Y., Oda, N., & Hosoda, S. (2002, December). Hyperviscoelasticity of epipharyngeal mucus may induce globus pharynges. *Annals of Otology, Rhinology and Laryngology, 111*(12 Pt. 1), 1116–1119.

Solyom, L., & Sookman, D. (1980). Fear of choking and its treatment. A behavioral approach. *Canadian Journal of Psychiatry, 25*(1), 30–34.

Steinhausen, H., Aster, M. V., Pfeiffer P., & Gobel, D. (1989). Comparative studies of conversion disorders in childhood and adolescents. *Journal of Child Psychology and Psychiatry, 30*, 615–621.

Sunku, B., Marino, R. V., & Sockolow, R. (2000, December). A primary care approach to pediatric gastroesophageal reflux. Review. *Journal of American Osteopathic Association, 100*(12 Suppl.), S11–5.

Thompson, M. (2002). The pediatric esophagus comes of age. *Journal of Pediatric Gastroenterology and Nutrition, 34*(Suppl. 1), 540–545.

Tokashiki, R., Yamaguchi, H., Nakamura, K., & Suzuki, M. (2002, October). Globus sensation caused by gastroesophageal reflux disease. *Auris, Nasus Larynx, 29*(4), 347–351.

Vandenplas, Y. (2000). Diagnosis and treatment of gastroesophageal reflux disease in infants and children. *Canadian Journal of Gastroenterology, 14*(Suppl. D), 26D–34D.

Vandenplas, Y., & Hegar, B. (2000). Diagnosis and treatment of gastroesophageal disease in infants and children. *Journal of Gastroenterology and Heptology, 15*, 593–603.

Vandenplas, Y., & Hassall, E. (2002). Pathophysiology of reflux disease. *Journal of Pediatric Disease and Nutrition, 35*, 119–136.

Whitehead, W. E., & Schuster, M. M. (1985). *Gastrointestinal disorders. Behavioral and physiological basis for treatment*. New York: Academic Press.

Williams, D. T., & Hirsch, G. (1988). The somatizing disorders: Somatoform disorders, factitious disorders and malingering. In C. J. Kestenbaum & D. T. Williams (Eds.), *Handbook of clinical assessment of children and adolescents* (pp. 743–768). New York: New York University Press.

Wilson, J. A. (1992, April). Globus sensation. *Clinical Otolaryngology and Allied Sciences, 17*(2), 105–106.

Wilson, J. A., Deary, I. J., & Maran, G. D. (1988). Is globus hystericus? *American Journal of Psychiatry, 153*, 335–339.

Wolff, S. (1973). Psychiatric disorders in childhood. In J. O. Forfar & J. C. Arneil (Eds.), *Textbook of paediatrics* (p. 1741). Edinborough: Churchill Livingstone.

Zeiter, D. K., & Hyams, J. (1999, January–February). Gastroesophageal reflux: Pathogenesis, diagnosis and treatment. *Allergy and Asthma Proceedings, 20*(1), 45–49.

Rumination and Cyclic Vomiting Syndrome | 5

RUMINATION

Rumination is characterized by voluntary regurgitation of stomach contents into the mouth, which are either expectorated or rechewed and reswallowed. The regurgitation is not caused by an associated gastrointestinal condition or other medical disorder. Rumination is a rare disorder that is most commonly seen in infants or persons who are developmentally disabled. It also occurs in children, adolescents, and adults with normal intelligence, albeit much less often. Insufficient awareness of the condition has led to underdiagnosis, with rumination frequently confused with bulimia nervosa, gastroesophageal reflux disease, and upper gastrointestinal motility disorders (Chial, Camilleri, Williams, Litzinger, & Perrault, 2003). When not appropriately diagnosed and treated, rumination can lead to serious complications, including weight loss, malnutrition, dental erosions, halitosis, electrolyte abnormalities, and significant functional disability (O'Brien, Bruce, & Camilleri, 1995).

The typical features of rumination have been described by Fleisher (1979) and O'Brien, Bruce, and Camilleri (1995) and summarized by Malcolm, Thumshirn, Camilleri, and Williams (1997). They include the following: (1) repetitive regurgitation of gastric contents occurring within minutes after a meal; (2) episodes often persist for 1 to 2 hours; (3) the regurgitated food consists of partially recognizable food; (4) the regurgitation is effortless or preceded by a sensation of belching immediately before the regurgitation or arrival of food in the pharynx; (5) usually, no retching or nausea precedes regurgitation; (6) patients have made a conscious decision about the regurgitated material once it is present in the oropharynx; and (7) rumination is typically a "meal in, meal out, day in, day out" behavior.

Currently, the diagnosis of rumination is based on symptom presentation, history, and the absence of disease (Malcolm et al., 1997; Rasquin-Weber et al., 1999). Standardized symptom-based criteria for child and adolescent rumination have yet to be developed. DSM-IV classifies "rumination disorder" as a disorder of infancy or early childhood, but does not specify criteria appropriate for older children and young adolescents. Similarly, the Rome II classification system (Rasquin-Weber et al., 1999) describes "infant rumination syndrome," which pertains to infants with symptom onset prior to 8 months of age, but does not include criteria for older age groups. To fill this void, Chial et al. (2003) proposed the following criteria: At least 6 weeks, which may not be consecutive, in the previous

81

12 months of recurrent regurgitation of recently ingested food that: (1) begins within 30 minutes of meal ingestion, (2) is associated with either reswallowing or expulsion of food, (3) stops within 90 minutes of onset or when regurgitant becomes acidic, (4) is not associated with mechanical obstruction, (5) does not respond to standard treatment for gastroesophageal reflux disease (i.e., medical therapy or lifestyle modification measures), and (6) is not associated with nocturnal symptoms. Acceptance of these or alternate diagnostic criteria will be important for providing clinicians with a standardized manner of identifying rumination. Moreover, consensus criteria will be essential for future research efforts examining the physiology and treatment of rumination.

Prevalence and Prognosis

Although there are no recent prevalence reports, existing studies suggest that rumination is not a common disorder (Singh, 1981; Whitehead & Schuster, 1985). Prevalence rates vary according to the population. Rumination occurs in 6% to 10% of institutionalized persons who are mentally retarded (Ball, Hendricksen, & Clayton, 1974; Singh, 1981), but is less common in infancy (Fleisher, 1979). It is reportedly underdiagnosed in children, adolescents, and adults with normal intelligence (Chial et al., 2003). Within this latter group, patients with bulimia nervosa have been found to be especially at risk, with prevalence rates of 17% to 20% (Fairburn & Cooper, 1984; O'Brien, Bruce, & Camilleri, 1995).

Among infants, the typical age of onset for rumination is between 3 and 12 months of age. In individuals with mental retardation, it may emerge later. The diagnosis is often delayed in children and adolescents with rumination beginning after infancy. In a study of patients ages 5 to 20 with rumination, Chial et al. (2003) found that the mean age at diagnosis was 15 years, with an average symptom duration before diagnosis of 2.2 years. The disorder often remits spontaneously, but, in severe cases, may be continuous. School and work absenteeism, hospitalization, and other features of functional disability may be significant (Chial et al., 2003).

Causes/Conceptualization

Theories of the etiology of rumination have focused on problems in the parent-child relationship or the reinforcing aspects of the ruminative act (Linscheid & Cunningham, 1977). Traditional psychodynamic explanations focus on disturbed and faulty mothering (e.g., maternal difficulties with comforting and nurturing), albeit rumination may actually develop from reciprocal interactions between the parent and the child. For example, the caregiver may become discouraged and alienated because of unsuccessful feeding experiences or the aversive odor of regurgitated food. As a result, appropriate comfort and nurturing are not provided. Behavioral theories posit that rumination is a learned behavior reinforced by the taste of the regurgitated food or the associated attention from adults (Linscheid, 1983). Over time, the act of rumination may be maintained by its self-stimulatory nature and become habitual.

Physiologically, relaxation of the lower esophageal sphincter (LES) reduces the physical barrier to regurgitation and appears to have a primary role in the process of rumination (Thumshirn et al., 1998). The specific mechanism by which gastric contents are regurgitated through the esophagus into the oropharynx remains unclear (Malcolm et al., 1997). Possible explanations include: (1) simultaneous relaxation of the LES at the time of increased intra-abdominal pressure, (2) learned voluntary relaxation of the LES that permits regurgitation (Smout & Breumelhof, 1990), and (3) learned adaptation of the belch reflex (O'Brien et al., 1995). With the latter, air swallowing is postulated to produce gastric distension, which leads to relaxation of the LES. When the upper esophageal sphincter relaxes, food is ejected into the mouth and expelled or reswallowed, depending on the social circumstances.

Clinical Evaluation

As noted, the clinical diagnosis of rumination is based on symptom presentation, history, and the absence of disease. Observation of the ruminative act is essential. It is important to note, however, that rumination may cease the moment the child notices an observer (Rasquin-Weber et al., 1999). Though some investigations (e.g., esophagogastroduodenoscopy, scintigraphic studies of gastric emptying, 24-hour esophageal pH testing) to rule out physical and organic causes may be warranted, patients often undergo unnecessary and expensive testing. Gastrointestinal manometry has been advocated as a diagnostic test for rumination because of evidence of a characteristic pattern of waves (Amarnath, Abell, & Malagelada, 1986). Chial et al. (2003), however, found that only 40% of their rumination patients had these characteristic waves. Their results suggest that with typical clinical features, gastrointestinal manometry may be unnecessary.

The focus of the psychosocial assessment is the parent-child relationship. Important areas for assessment include parental feelings toward self and the child, parental ability to recognize and respond sensitively to the child's physical and emotional needs, life stress, and psychological symptoms. Observation of aversive parent-child interactions supports the diagnosis of rumination. From a behavioral perspective, identification of antecedents and potentially reinforcing consequences is important. The social attention elicited by the ruminative act may serve as a strong reinforcer that maintains or strengthens the behavior. As noted earlier, ruminative behavior may become self-stimulatory and habitual in nature. Attention to the possible function that rumination serves is essential for understanding and treating the disorder. For example, a child's rumination may be negatively reinforced because it allows avoidance of more aversive situations/circumstances.

Treatment

Treatment efforts are typically directed toward enhancing the parent-child relationship. Improving the caregiver's ability to recognize and respond appropriately to the child's needs is often an important component of therapy. Instruction in parent-child interaction skills, support and direct assistance, individual psychotherapy, or medication for depression or other emotional difficulties may be warranted.

Behaviorally, aversive or punishment strategies (e.g., squirting lemon juice into the child's mouth, excluding the child from social interaction) have been utilized for rumination that appears reinforced by the taste of regurgitated food or associated attention from adults. Though aversive treatment methods may not lead to adverse side effects (Linscheid, 1983), such techniques have been associated with increases in other self-stimulatory behaviors following suppression of rumination (Malcolm et al., 1997). Ethical issues need to be carefully evaluated when considering the use of these techniques.

Nonaversive behavioral treatments are appropriate for children, adolescents, as well as adults with normal intelligence. Among the strategies that have been found effective are thorough explanation of the condition, strong encouragement not to vomit, progressive muscle relaxation, and biofeedback to relax the stomach muscles before and after eating (Malcolm et al., 1997). Wagaman, Williams, and Camilleri (1998) presented a case report of a simplified habit-reversal approach for the treatment of rumination in a 6-year-old girl of normal intelligence. The girl presented with a 1-year history of rumination, and, at her initial evaluation, reported ruminating 12 times in approximately 40 minutes. The habit-reversal approach consisted of awareness training, the use of incompatible behavior (diaphragmatic breathing), and social support from the girl's parents. After implementation of a reinforcement program for practicing breathing exercises, the rumination episodes decreased. The frequency of days without rumination gradually increased until rumination was not reported after day 107. The mother did not report smelling the odor of rumination on the child's breath at day 21. Chial et al. (2003) reported that the vast majority of their rumination patients had significant symptom improvement or resolution following a similar habit reversal approach. Participants in their study were 46 children and adolescents, ranging in age from 5 to 20. Symptoms resolved in 16 (29.6%) and improved in 30 (55.5%). Overall, a positive impact in symptoms was noted in 85.1%.

CYCLIC VOMITING SYNDROME

Cyclic vomiting syndrome (CVS) is characterized by recurrent, stereotypical episodes of severe nausea and vomiting lasting hours to days, separated by symptom-free intervals. As many as 70 episodes of vomiting are experienced per year, with an average of 9 to 12 a year (Forbes, 1999). These episodes typically last from 1 to 4 days but can last as long as 10 days. The intervals between attacks may be fairly regular or sporadic. Within an individual, episodes tend to be similar in terms of time of onset, intensity, duration, frequency, associated symptoms, and signs (Fleisher & Matar, 1993). Episodes usually begin during the night or early morning, with vomiting reaching its highest intensity during the first hours (Pfau & Li, 1996). Accompanying signs and symptoms include photophobia, headache, fever, motion sickness, and abdominal pain.

Each CVS episode typically progresses through four phases: prodrome, episode, recovery, and the symptom-free interval. The prodrome signals that an episode of nausea and vomiting is forthcoming. This phase is characterized by abdominal pain and can last from just a few minutes to several hours. Occasionally, taking medicine during the prodrome can abort an approaching episode. At other times, a person may wake in the morning and begin vomiting with little to no warning. The episode phase consists of nausea and vomiting; inability to eat, drink, or take medicine without vomiting; pallor; and exhaustion. Recovery begins when the nausea and vomiting ends. Appetite, healthy color, and energy then return. The symptom-free interval is the period between episodes when no symptoms are present.

Rome II diagnostic criteria for CVS include the following: (1) a history of three or more periods of intense, acute nausea, and unremitting vomiting lasting hours to days, with intervening symptom-free intervals, lasting weeks to months, and (2) there is no metabolic, gastrointestinal, or central nervous system structural or biochemical disease (Rasquin-Weber et al., 1999). An alternate set of diagnostic criteria were generated at the International Scientific Symposium on Cyclic Vomiting Syndrome held at St. Bartholomew's Hospital in London, U.K., in 1994. These criteria defined essential and supportive elements for the diagnosis. Essential criteria include: (1) recurrent, severe, discrete episodes of vomiting; (2) varying intervals of normal health between episodes; (3) duration of vomiting episodes from hours to days; and (4) no apparent cause of vomiting with negative laboratory, radiographic, and endoscopic results. Supportive criteria are: (1) vomiting pattern is stereotypical, and each episode is similar as to time of onset, intensity, duration, frequency, and associated symptoms within an individual; (2) vomiting pattern is self-limited, and episodes resolve spontaneously if left untreated; (3) associated symptoms include nausea, abdominal pain, headache, motion sickness, and lethargy; and (4) associated signs include fever, pallor, diarrhea, dehydration, excess salivation, and social withdrawal.

It is important to note that the terms CVS and abdominal migraine have often been used interchangeably because of the overlap in clinical presentation (Sundaram & Li, 2002). Except for vomiting, the primary characteristics of abdominal migraine are similar to those of CVS: recurrent, stereotypical episodes of severe abdominal pain; intervening symptom-free intervals; autonomic nervous system symptoms (e.g., lethargy, pallor); and a family history of migraine headaches. When both abdominal pain and vomiting are present, the predominant symptom is used as the primary label. Moreover, similarities between CVS and not only abdominal migraines but also migraine headaches suggest that CVS may be a migraine variant. As discussed later, the type of migraine manifested may reflect a developmental progression (Abu-Arafeh & Russell, 1995; Sundaram & Li, 2002). It remains unclear why some children develop CVS and not other migraine syndromes.

Prevalence and Prognosis

Population-based studies suggest that the prevalence of CVS is approximately 2%. For example, epidemiological data reported by Cullen and MacDonald (1963) estimated the prevalence of "periodic" vomiting in western Australia to be 2.3%. Abu-Arafeh and Russell (1995) reported a prevalence of 1.9% in school-age children in Aberdeen, Scotland. Females show a slight predominance over males (11:9) (Li, Murray, Heitlinger, Robbins, & Hayes, 1999). CVS occurs from infancy throughout adulthood, but the median age of onset is 5.2 years (Li & Balint, 2000). Prakash, Staiano, Rothbaum, & Clouse (2001) reported that many of the characteristics of CVS are similar irrespective of age of onset. Duration of episodes, however, was reported to increase with age, up to 20 years.

According to Sundaram and Li (2002), CVS typically lasts an average of 2.5 to 5.5 years, resolving in late childhood or early adolescence. Some individuals, however, continue to be symptomatic through adulthood. In a study of the medium-term prognosis of CVS, Dignan, Symon, Abu-Arafeh, and Russell (2001) found that 50% of affected persons had continuing CVS or migraine headaches, whereas the remainder were currently asymptomatic. Existing prognostic data suggest that CVS may be an age-dependent manifestation of migraines. The typical progression is that CVS progresses to abdominal migraines and then to migraine headaches (Sundaram & Li, 2002). Abu-Arafeh and Russell (1995) reported that the mean ages of children with CVS, abdominal migraines, and migraine headaches were 5.3, 10.3, and 11.5 years, respectively. Sundaram and Li (2002) have observed a similar progression and found that nearly one third of their patients develop migraines after resolution of CVS. He and his colleagues predicted that nearly 60% of persons affected by CVS eventually develop migraines.

Causes/Conceptualization

The cause of CVS is not clear. Various physiological factors have been investigated, including migraine-related mechanisms and neuronal hyperexcitability (Sundaram & Li, 2002). Sympathetic hyperresponsivity and autonomic dysfunction also appear to contribute to CVS (Gordan, 1994) and are thought to mediate related symptoms such as fever, pallor, diarrhea, and salivation. Another contributor is stress activation of the hypothalamic-pituitary-adrenal axis, which can also trigger CVS episodes (Li et al., 1999; Li & Fleisher, 1999) To date, no all-encompassing etiological model exists to integrate these physiological contributors with the psychosocial variables associated with CVS. The broad biopsychosocial model of functional gastrointestinal disorders, with its attention to interactions between physiological and psychosocial factors via various brain-gut mechanisms, provides a basic framework for understanding and treating cyclic vomiting.

The older psychological literature characterized individuals with CVS as manifesting a tendency toward anxiety and excitability and blamed the disorder on disturbed relationships with parents (Forbes, 1999). Seventy-six percent of parents of children with CVS described their children as having one or more of the following traits: competitive, perfectionistic, high-achieving, aggressive, strong-willed, moralistic, caring, and enthusiastic (Fleisher & Matar, 1993). More recent research (Forbes, Withers, Silburn, & McKelvey, 1999; Withers, Silburn, & Forbes, 1998) found that children with CVS had more clinically significant scores on the Child Behavior Checklist (CBCL) than healthy children. Children with CVS manifested a tendency toward anxiety, depression, and other internalizing symptoms. CVS can be incapacitating and can result in considerable functional impairment, including poor school attendance. Sixty percent of children with CVS miss more than 10 school days a year because of vomiting, and 15% missed more than a month of school (Withers et al., 1998).

Most families are able to identify events that appear to precipitate or trigger a patient's vomiting episode (Cullen & McDonald, 1983; Withers et al., 1998; Li & Fleisher, 1999; Hoyt, & Stickler, 1960). The most common trigger is an infection (41%), particularly chronic sinusitis. Another common trigger, often seen in children, is emotional stress or excitement (34%), both positive (e.g., birthday, vacation) and negative. Eating certain foods, such as chocolate, cheese, and monosodium glutamate (MSG), is another precipitant. Lack of sleep (18%), menstruation (13%), and motion sickness (13%) can also trigger episodes.

Clinical Evaluation

Diagnosis of CVS is difficult and is made by a review of history, physical examination, and studies to rule out other possible causes of vomiting. The numerous medical explanations for vomiting, as well as the complications associated with severe vomiting, underscore the importance of an accurate diagnosis. Differential diagnosis should include the multiple gastrointestinal, central nervous system, autonomic nervous system, urinary tract, or endocrine and metabolic disorders that may cause nausea and vomiting (Forbes, 1999; Sundaram & Li, 2002). Among the common disorders presenting with recurrent vomiting are brain stem tumors, obstructive uropathy, peptic disease, recurrent pancreatitis, intermittent bowel obstruction, intestinal pseudo-obstruction, and familial dysautonomia (Fleisher, 1994; Forbes, 1999; Rasquin-Weber et al., 1999). Endocrine and metabolic diseases that mimic cyclic vomiting include diabetic ketoacidosis, adrenal insufficiency, pheochromcytoma, urea cycle defects, medium-chain acyl-CoA dehyrogenase deficiency, organic academias, and porphyria. CVS workup is individualized and guided by patient's symptom presentation. Workup may include blood studies, urine studies, stool studies, and imaging studies (Fleisher, 1994; Forbes, 1999).

The psychological evaluation aids in differential diagnosis and is important for assessing: (1) the extent to which stress and emotional factors contribute to vomiting and (2) the effectiveness of child and familial coping efforts. Among the psychological disorders to be considered in the differential diagnosis are Munchausen's syndrome by proxy, anxiety, depression, anorexia nervosa, and bulimia nervosa (Fleisher, 1999; Sundaram & Li, 2002). Diaries of the antecedents, symptoms, and consequences of CVS episodes may reveal precipitants, associated features, and maladaptive responses that are not evident (Jellinek, 1997). Special attention should be given to changes in family life in response to the child's perceived needs, "vulnerable child" status for the child, or an immature or overly intense parent-child relationship (Jellinek, 1997). These parental and familial factors may inadvertently reinforce or maintain cyclic vomiting. For example, extra attention for the child with CVS may lead to continued vomiting.

Treatment

To date, no specific cure for CVS exists. Medical management is individualized and guided by the phase of the episode. Treatment of the acute cyclic vomiting episode includes attempts to shorten the episode, treat the symptoms, and minimize associated complications (Forbes, 1999). Prevention of future episodes requires a collaborative effort between the patient, family, and health care providers. Much trial and error may be involved in establishing the most effective treatment/prevention plan.

During the prodrome, abortive medications, such as ondansetron (Zofran), erythromycin (E.E.S., Eryc, E-Mycin, Erythrocin), and ibuprofen, may be useful prior to the onset of nausea (Rasquin-Weber et al., 1999). Once the episode begins, treatment is generally supportive. Induction of sleep has long been considered beneficial in controlling vomiting episodes (Fleisher, 1994). A dark, quiet environment with few interventions and little disturbance is essential. Lorazepam (Ativan), with its anxiolytic, sedative, and antiemetic effects, has been used to suppress or shorten episodes of cyclic vomiting (Puls, 1990). According to Li (2000), intravenous fluid replacement can diminish the severity of vomiting episodes by 42%. Though oral intake is typically limited to minimize vomiting, some patients prefer large volumes of liquid during episodes as it may temporarily decrease their nausea (Fleisher, 1995). An oral acid-inhibiting drug to protect esophageal mucosa and dental enamel may also be helpful (Rasquin-Weber et al., 1999).

During the recovery phase, fluid and electrolyte replacement is essential. Intravenous fluids and 10% dextrose help prevent dehydration and ketosis

(Forbes, 1999). Intense hunger is common following cyclic vomiting episodes. Though some individuals are able to resume an unrestricted diet, others experience a recurrence of symptoms after eating their first postepisodic meal. For those with these recurrences, limiting oral intake to isotonic or hypotonic nutrient liquids in the first day or two has been recommended (Fleisher, 1994).

During the symptom-free interval, medications used for migraine prophylaxis, such as propranolol (Inderal), amitriptyline (Elavil), and cyproheptadine (Periactin), may be helpful. One to 2-month trials of these medications may be particularly useful for patients whose episodes are frequent and enduring. Li (1996) recommended prophylactic therapy for patients who have episodes once per month or if episodes last at least 3 days. For those with a positive family history of migraines, there is a high response rate (80%) to antimigraine medications (Li & Bailint, 2000). When the child is symptom free, other medical problems (e.g., sinus problems, allergies) causing episodes should be treated. In some instances, avoidance of identified dietary triggers such as chocolate and cheese may prevent episodes without the use of medication (Li & Balint, 2000).

The symptom-free interval is also appropriate for identification and treatment of factors that may predispose to or trigger episodes (e.g., family therapy to reduce emotional stress). Diaries of the antecedents, symptoms, and consequences of symptoms may reveal precipitating factors, maladaptive coping efforts, and other associated factors. For those with a tendency toward anxiety, relaxation training and biofeedback may enhance physiological control, contributing to a decrease in the frequency and severity of episodes (Jellinek, 1997).

Clinically, the importance of an understanding, respectful, and knowledgeable clinician cannot be overstated (Forbes, 1999). The diagnosis of CVS is often delayed or unrecognized, leading to despair, anger, and a loss of a sense of well-being. Consultation with a sympathetic gastroenterologist without drug therapy has been found to reduce the frequency of cyclic vomiting episodes as much as 70%, revealing a strong placebo effect (Li, 2000). Mental health support and treatment assists families in handling the physical and emotional stressors associated with CVS. To that end, the Cyclic Vomiting Syndrome Association (CVSA) is an excellent resource for interparent support as well as education for both families and professionals. (Their mailing address is CVSA, 3585 Cedar Hill Rd, N.W., Canal Winchester, OH 43110, and their website is located at www.cvsaonline.org.)

REFERENCES

Abu-Arafeh, I., & Russell, G. (1995). Prevalence and clinical features of abdominal migraine compared to those of migraine headache. *Archives of Diseases in Childhood, 72,* 413–417.
Amarnath, R. P., Abell, T. L., & Malagelada, J. R. (1986). The rumination syndrome in adults: A characteristic manometric pattern. *Annals of Internal Medicine, 105,* 513–518.

American Psychiatric Association. (1994). *Diagnostic and statistical manual of mental disorders* (4th ed.). Washington, DC: American Psychiatric Association.

Ball, R. S., Hendricksen, H., & Clayton, J. (1974). A special feeding technique for chronic regurgitation. *American Journal of Mental Deficiency, 78*, 486–493.

Battistella, P. A., Carra, S., Zaninotto, Ruffilli, R., & Da Dalt, L. (1992). Pupillary reactivity in children with recurrent abdominal pain. *Headache, 32*, 105–107.

Browne, S. E. (1997). Brief hypnotherapy with passive children. *Contemporary Hypnosis, 14*, 59–62.

Bursch, B. (1999). Pain-Associated Disability Syndrome. In P. E. Hyman (Ed.), *Pediatric functional gastrointestinal disorders* (pp. 8.1-8.14). New York: Academic Professional Information Services.

Bursch B., Walco, G. A., & Zeltzer, L. (1998). Clinical assessment and management of chronic pain and pain-associated disability syndrome. *Journal of Developmental and Behavioral Pediatrics, 195*, 45–53.

Chial, H. J., Camilleri, M., Williams, D. E., Litzinger, K., & Perrault, J. (2003). Rumination syndrome in children and adolescents: Diagnosis, treatment, and prognosis. *Pediatrics, 111*, 158–162.

Coderre, T. J., Katz, J., Vaccarino, A. L., & Melzack, R. (1993). Contribution of central neuroplasticity to pathological pain: Review of clinical and experimental evidence. *Pain, 52*, 259–285.

Connor-Smith, J. K., Compas, B. E., Wadsworth, M. E., Thomson, A. H., & Saltzman, H. (2000). Responses to stress in adolescence: Measurement of coping and involuntary stress responses. *Journal of Consulting and Clinical Psychology, 68*, 976–992.

Cullen, K. J., & McDonald, W. B. (1963). The periodic syndrome: Its nature and prevalence. *Medical Journal of Australia, 167*–173.

Dignan, F., Symon D. N. K., AbuArafeh, I., & Russell, G. (2001). The prognosis of cyclical vomiting syndrome. *Archives of Disease in Childhood, 84*, 55–57.

Fairburn, C. G., & Cooper, P. J. (1984). Rumination in bulimia nervosa. *British Medical Journal, 288*, 826–827.

Feuerstein, M., Barr, R.G., Francoeur, R. E., Houle, M., & Rafman, S. (1982). Potential biobehavioral mechanisms of recurrent abdominal pain in children. *Pain, 13*, 287–298.

Fleisher, D. R. (1979). Infant rumination syndrome. *American Journal of Diseases in Children, 133*, 266–269.

Fleisher, D. R. (1994). Cyclic vomiting. In P. Hyman (Ed.), *Pediatric Gastrointestinal Motility Disorders* (pp. 89–104). New York: Academy Professional Information Services, Inc.

Fleisher, D. R. (1995). Management of cyclic vomiting syndrome. *Journal of Pediatric Gastroenterology and Nutrition, 21*, S52–S56.

Fleisher, D. R., & Matar, M. (1993). The cyclic vomiting syndrome: A report of 71 cases and a literature review. *Journal of Pediatric Gastroenterology, 17*, 361–369.

Forbes, D. (1999). Cyclic vomiting syndrome. In P. E. Hyman (Ed.), *Pediatric functional gastrointestinal disorders* (pp. 5.1–5.12). New York: Academy Professional Information Services.

Forbes, D., Withers, G., Silburn, S., & McKelvey, R. (1999). Psychological and social characteristics and precipitants of vomiting in children with cyclic vomiting syndrome. *Digestive Diseases and Sciences, 44 (8)*, 19S–22S.

Gordan, N. (1994). Recurrent vomiting in childhood, especially of neurological origin. *Developmental Medicine Clinics, 36*, 463–467.

Gragg, R. A., Rapoff, M. A., Danovsky, M. B., Lindsley, C. B., Varni, J. W., Waldron, S. A., & Bernstein, B. H. (1996). Assessing chronic musculoskeletal pain associated with rheumatic disease: Further validation of the Pediatric Pain Questionnaire. *Journal of Pediatric Psychology, 24*, 115–127.

Hoyt, C., & Stickler, G. (1960). A study of 44 children with the syndrome of recurrent (cyclic) vomiting. *Pediatrics, 25*, 775–780.

Hyman, P. E. (Ed.) (1999). *Pediatric functional gastrointestinal disorders*. New York: Academic Professional Information Services.

Kline, R. M., Kline, J. J., Di Palma, J., & Barbero, G. J. (2001). Enteric-coated, pH dependent peppermint oil capsules for the treatment of irritable bowel syndrome in children. *Journal of Pediatrics, 138,* 125–128.

Kopel, F. B., Kim, I. C., & Barbero, G. J. (1967). Comparison of rectosigmoid motility in normal children, children with recurrent abdominal pain, and children with ulcerative colitis. *Pediatrics, 39,* 539–545.

Jellinek, M. S. (1997). Comment on cyclic vomiting. *Journal of Developmental and Behavioral Pediatrics, 18,* 269.

Li, Bu. (2000). Current treatment of cyclic vomiting syndrome. *Current Treatment Options in Gastroenterology, 3,* 395–402.

Li, Bu., & Balint, J. P. (2000). Cyclic vomiting syndrome: Evolution in our understanding of a brain-gut disorder. *Advances in Pediatrics, 47,* 117–160.

Li, Bu., & Fleisher, D. R. (1999). Cyclic vomiting syndrome: Features to be explained by a patho-physiological model. *Digestive Diseases and Sciences, 44*(8), 13S–18S.

Li, Bu., Murray, R. D., Heitlinger, L. A., Robbins, J. L., & Hayes, J. R. (1999). Is cyclic vomiting syndrome related to migraine? *Journal of Pediatrics, 134,* 533–535.

Linscheid, T. R. (1983). Eating problems in children. In C. E. Walker & M. C. Roberts (Eds.), *Handbook of clinical child psychology* (pp. 616–639). New York: Wiley.

Linscheid, T. R., & Cunningham, C. E. (1977). A controlled demonstration of the effectiveness of electric shock in the elimination of chronic infant rumination. *Journal of Applied Behavior Analysis, 10,* 500.

Malcolm, A., Thumshirn, M. B., Camilleri, M., & Williams, D. E. (1997). Rumination syndrome. *Mayo Clinic Proceedings, 72,* 646–652.

Mayer, E. A. (1993). Functional bowel disorders and the visceral hyperalgesia hypothesis. In. E. A. Meyers & H. E. Raybould (Eds.), *Basic and clinical aspects of chronic abdominal pain* (pp. 3–28). New York: Elsevier.

O'Brien, M. D., Bruce, B. K., & Camilleri, M. (1995). The rumination syndrome: Clinical features rather than manometiric diagnosis. *Gastroenterology, 108,* 1024–1029.

Pfau, B. T., & Li, B. U. K. (1996). Differentiating cyclic from chronic vomiting patterns in children—quantitative criteria and diagnostic implications. *Pediatrics, 97,* 367–368.

Prakash, C., Staiano, A., Rothbaum, R. J., & Clouse, R. E. (2001). Similarities in cyclic vomiting syndrome across age groups. *American Journal of Gastroenterology, 96,* 684–688.

Puls, L. (1990). A recurrent vomiting syndrome in children. *Contemporary Pediatrics,* 8–11.

Rasquin-Weber, A., Hyman, P. E., Cucchiara, S., Fleisher, D. R., Hyams, J. S., Milla, P. J. et al. (1999). Childhood functional gastrointestinal disorders. *Gut, 45*(Suppl. 2), 1160–1168.

Risser, A. L., & Mazur, L. J. (1993). Use of folk remedies in a Hispanic population. *Archives of Pediatric and Adolescent Medicine, 149,* 978–981.

Rubin, L. S., Barbero, G. J., & Sibinga, M. S. (1967). Pupillary reactivity in children with recurrent abdominal pain. *Psychosomatic Medicine, 29,* 111–120.

Sanders, M. R., Patel, R. K., & Woolford, H. H. (1993). *Treatment of recurrent abdominal pain: A therapist's manual.* Unpublished manuscript.

Singh, N. N. (1981). Rumination. *International Review of Research in Mental Retardation, 10,* 139–182.

Sokel, B., Devane, S., & Bentovim, A. (1991). Getting better with honor: Individualized relaxation/self-hypnosis techniques for control of recalcitrant abdominal pain in children. *Family Systems Medicine, 9,* 83–91.

Smout, A. J., & Breumelhof, R. (1990). Voluntary induction of transient lower esophageal sphincter relaxations in an adult patient with the rumination syndrome. *American Journal of Gastroenterology, 85,* 1621–1625.

Sundaram, S., & Li, Bu. (2002). Cyclic vomiting syndrome. *http://www.medicine.com/ped/topic2910.htm*

Thumshirn, M., Camilleri, M. C., Hanson, R. B., Williams, D. E., Schei, A. J., & Kammer, P. P. (1998). Gastric mechanosensory and lower esophageal sphincter function in rumination syndrome. *American Journal of Physiology, 275,* G314–G321.

Turner, K. M. T., Woolford, H. H., & Sanders, M. R. (1993). *Pain management: A manual to help you manage your pain*. Unpublished manuscript.

Van Slyke, D. A. (2000). *Illness Behavior Encouragement Scales-Revised*. Unpublished manuscript.

Wagaman, J. R., Williams, D. E., & Camilleri, M. (1998). Behavioral intervention for the treatment of rumination. *Journal of Pediatric Gastroenterology and Nutrition, 27*, 596–598.

Walker, L. S., & Greene, J. W. (1991b). The Functional Disability Inventory: Measuring a neglected dimension of child health status. *Journal of Pediatric Psychology, 16*, 39–58.

Walker, L. S., Garber, J., & Green, J. W. (1993). Psychosocial correlates of recurrent childhood pain: A comparison of pediatric patients with recurrent abdominal pain, organic illness, and psychiatric disorders. *Journal of Abnormal Psychology, 102*, 248–258.

Wang, X. M. (1988). Electroimpulse acupuncture treatment of 110 cases of abdominal pain as a sequela of abdominal surgery. *Journal of Traditional Chinese Medicine, 8*, 269–270.

Whitehead, W. E., & Schuster, M. M. (1985). Rumination syndrome, vomiting, aerophagia, and belching. In W. E. Whitehead & M. M. Schuster (Eds.), *Gastrointestinal disorders: Behavioral and physiological basis for treatment* (pp. 67–90). Orlando, FL: Academic Press.

Withers, G. D., Silburn, S. R., & Forbes, D. A. (1998). Cyclic vomiting syndrome: A descriptive analysis of symptoms, precipitants, aetiology, and treatment. *Acta Paediatrica, 87*, 272–277.

Yanhua, S., & Sumei, Y. (2000). The treatment of 86 cases of epigastric and abdominal pain by scalp acupuncture. *Journal of Chinese Medicine, 62*, 27–29.

Recurrent Abdominal Pain | 6

The term *recurrent abdominal pain* (RAP) has been used and defined in various ways over time. Almost every paper or presentation on RAP, however, begins with a reference to Apley's criteria (Apley, 1975; Apley & Hale, 1973). According to Apley, RAP is characterized by three or more episodes of abdominal pain that occur over at least 3 months and are severe enough to interfere with activities, such as school attendance and performance, social activities, and participation in sports and extracurricular activities. Clinically, these episodes are characterized by vague abdominal pain that is dull or crampy, is poorly localized or periumbilical, and persists for less than 1 hour (Frazer & Rappaport, 1999). The pain frequently presents with nausea, vomiting, and other signs of autonomic arousal (Apley, 1975).

Though the term RAP is most often used to refer to functional abdominal pain, Apley's original description is broad and does not have specific etiological implications. The majority of children with RAP do not have a specific physical disorder or organic disease. Most investigators report that only 5% to 10% of affected children have an organic cause for their pain (Apley, 1975; Apley & Hale, 1958). Advances in medical diagnostics, however, have led to an increase in the identification of organic causes (Hyams, Burke, Davis, Rzepsaki, & Andrulonis, 1996), suggesting that past figures may somewhat underestimate the prevalence of organically caused pain (El-Matary, Spray & Sandhu, 2004).

Apley's criteria have recently been criticized for being ambiguous and allowing for both nonorganic and organic causes (Von Baeyer & Walker, 1999), and their continued use has been discouraged. Acknowledging this, Von Baeyer and Walker (1999) proposed a two-stage approach to classification of RAP. The first stage of classification involves a decision as to whether a child meets broad RAP criteria. Assignment at this stage requires that a child's clinical presentation be consistent with Apley's temporal and severity criteria for RAP (i.e., three or more pain episodes in at least 3 months, functional impairment). At the second stage, RAP subgroups are identified on the basis of medical findings and other symptoms. Examples include RAP with constipation, RAP with peptic ulcer, RAP without identified etiology, and RAP with constipation and depression. Another system for classifying functional (i.e., not organically caused) abdominal pain was proposed by the pediatric gastroenterology multinational Rome Working Team (Rasquin-Weber et al., 1999). They delineated five diagnostic categories, including functional dyspepsia, irritable bowel syndrome

(IBS), functional abdominal pain, abdominal migraine, and aerophagia, and presented specific symptom-based criteria for each.

Clearly, an important priority for future investigations is examination of the reliability and validity of the above mentioned or other systems for classifying RAP. Refinement in our identification and categorization of RAP will increase our understanding of its various subtypes and assist in the development of targeted treatment strategies. At present, the majority of RAP research tends to utilize Apley's criteria and excludes children with a presumed organic basis for their pain. Unless otherwise specified, the references cited in the remainder of this chapter describe children who meet these criteria and have no physical or organic basis for their pain.

EPIDEMIOLOGY

Studies of the prevalence of RAP have found disparate results, with rates ranging from 9% to almost 25% (Apley & Naish, 1958; Oster, 1972). Inconsistent use of diagnostic criteria and characteristics of the population being sampled (e.g., age, gender) contribute to the conflicting findings. In general, population-based studies suggest that RAP is experienced by 10% to 15% of school-age children (Apley, 1975; Apley & Naish, 1958) and almost 20% of middle school and high school students (Hyams et al., 1996). As children grow older, the incidence of RAP appears to decrease in boys but not girls (Apley & Naish, 1958; Stickler & Murphy, 1979). Clinically, RAP often coexists with other somatic symptoms, such as chronic headache, with rates of comorbidity ranging from 14% to 90% (Hodges, Kline, Barbero, & Flanery, 1985; Scharff, 1997).

Investigations of the prognosis for RAP have also yielded conflicting findings. Differences in the severity of symptoms, nature of treatment, or length of follow-up may explain the discrepancies in these findings. Stickler and Murphy (1979) reported that 76% of their RAP sample no longer exhibited symptoms at a minimum follow-up of 5 years. Almost one-fourth failed to resolve their abdominal pain. Of the 76% who no longer had pain, 48% manifested other psychosomatic or physical complaints. The nature or extent of treatment that these patients received was not specified. Apley and Hale (1973) reported that 64% of children treated with reassurance had no abdominal pain at 10 to 14 year follow-up. Over one-third had continuing abdominal pains. Among the 64% without pain, 52% had other physical complaints, particularly headaches. Sixty percent of untreated children in their sample had no abdominal pain at follow-up. Long-term follow-up of children hospitalized for RAP (as late as 28 to 30 years after) has indicated that a smaller number, between 30% and 47%, will have complete resolution of their symptoms (Apley, 1959; Christensen & Mortensen, 1975). In a more recent study, Stordal, Nygaard and Bensten (2005) found that former RAP patients reported RAP, headache, and school absence more frequently than controls at a five-year follow-up. A high proportion of children referred with RAP had persistent symptoms, with more headache and school absence than controls.

ETIOLOGY/CONCEPTUAL MODELS

In the four decades since Apley's seminal research, conceptual models of RAP have evolved and become more complex. Walker (1999b) identified three distinct periods in this evolution. Studies conducted before the 1980s were characterized by a dualistic view of abdominal pain. When no organic etiology was identified, abdominal pain was assumed to be psychogenic. In the 1980s, the focus of research shifted to nonorganic causes of RAP, including a host of psychosocial factors. Conceptual models emerging in this decade were increasingly multivariate in nature. They recognized that the cause of RAP may be neither organic nor psychogenic, but possibly a function of normal (i.e., nonpathological) biological mechanisms. In the 1990s, the research focus shifted to the identification of individual differences among children with RAP and the interactive effects between contributing factors. As we enter the 21st century, conceptual models of RAP are multivariate and acknowledge the contributions of a variety of biological, psychological, and social factors. The following are two recently developed models that exemplify current biopsychosocial conceptualizations of RAP.

The Rome Group proposed a broad biopsychosocial conceptualization that applies to the etiology and course of a wide range of functional GI disorders, including childhood functional abdominal pain (Drossman, 2000). This model presumes that a child's condition is a function of multiple interacting determinants, including early life factors (e.g., genetic predisposition, environmental factors), physiological factors (e.g., motility, sensation), psychosocial factors (e.g., life stress, psychological state, coping, social support), and interactions between physiological and psychological factors via the central nervous system/enteric nervous system axis (see Figure 6.1). According to this model, a child with abdominal pain but with no psychosocial problems as well as good coping skills and social support will have a better outcome than the child with pain as well as coexisting emotional difficulties, high life stress, and limited support. The child's clinical outcome (e.g., daily function, quality of life) will, in turn, affect the severity of the disorder.

Walker (1999b) developed a conceptual model focusing specifically on the role of psychosocial factors in the course of RAP in middle childhood. This model proposes the psychosocial mechanisms that lead some children with RAP to develop sick role behavior (e.g., frequent somatic complaints, activity restrictions, and dependence on caretakers), while others do not (see Figure 6.2). According to the model, the amount of activity restriction

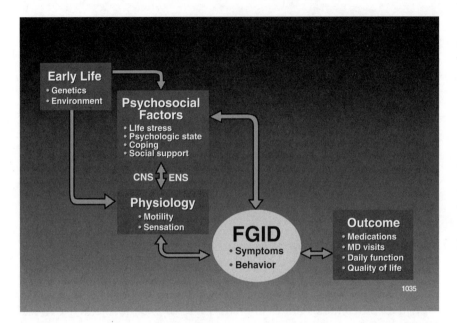

FIGURE 6.1. A biophychosocial conceptualization of the pathogenesis and clinical expression of the functional GI disorders (Drossman, 2000). (Reproduced by permission of CONF/NASPGHAN from the CME CD-ROM *Pediatric Gastroesophageal Reflux Disease, Evaluation and Management,* developed by the Children's Digestive Health and Nutrition Foundation and the North American Society for Pediatric Gastroenterology, Hepatology and Nutrition.)

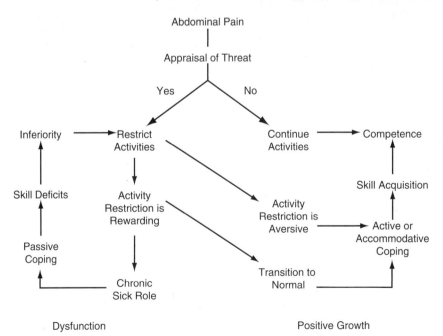

FIGURE 6.2. The course of pain: Cycles of dysfunction versus positive growth (Walker, 1999b).

associated with abdominal pain and the extent to which this restriction is perceived as rewarding or aversive play significant roles in determining whether or not pain results in functional disability.

PHYSIOLOGICAL FEATURES

More than 100 organic causes of abdominal pain have been identified in children and adolescents (Levine & Rappaport, 1984). These causes include obstruction of the intestinal tract, reactions to infection, inflammations, or ulcer, spinal disease, allergic reactions, metabolic disorders, and epilepsy. In cases with a specific etiology, there are usually "red flags" on history or examination that lead to the proper medical diagnosis (Frazer & Rappaport, 1999). As noted, however, a specific organic cause is identified in only a small number of children with RAP. As such, the majority of research on physical or organic features has centered on nonpathological biological mechanisms.

A number of studies have investigated various indices of autonomic nervous system (ANS) functioning (e.g., pupillary reactivity, cold presor response) in children with RAP (e.g., Battistella, Carra, Zaninotto, Ruffilli, & Da Dalt, 1992; Feuerstein, Barr, Franoeur, Houle, & Rafman, 1982; Kopel, Kim, & Barbero, 1967; Rubin, Barbero, & Sabenga, 1967). These investigations have examined two possibilities: (1) children with RAP are autonomically hypersensitive to stressors in ways that adversely impact gastrointestinal functioning and lead to abdominal pain and (2) RAP children have slow autonomic recovery following exposure to stress. The results of these studies have been conflicting and, to date, no specific ANS dysfunction has been identified and no clear etiologic role for ANS instability has been established.

Altered gastrointestinal motility has been another focus for physiological research. The role of motility disturbance has been clearly established in other gastrointestinal disorders, like diarrhea and constipation. For example, in the case of diarrhea, muscle contractions in the bowel are stronger and more frequent, and the feces move through the colon too quickly. There is not enough time to remove water from the feces, and the stools are loose and watery. Motility studies of children with RAP have not been as definitive as those of other gastrointestinal disorders. No specific pattern of altered motility has been found in patients with RAP. Moreover, recent data have shown a poor correlation between gastrointestinal motility and pain (Youseff & DiLorenzo, 2001).

Abnormalities in visceral sensation have been well documented in adult studies (Coderre et al., 1993; Mayer, 1993) and may also play a role in children. Existing research suggests that children with RAP may have abnormal perception of gastrointestinal physiological events and a lower threshold for pain. Similarly, Duarte, Goulart, and Penna (2001) reported that pain thresholds were reduced in all body regions of children with RAP. The reduced pain threshold seen in these children is hypothesized to be related to biochemical changes in the afferent neurons of the central and enteric nervous systems and can be influenced by cognitive processes (e.g., emotions, memories) or extrinsic sensations (e.g., smell).

PSYCHOLOGICAL FEATURES

Studies of the psychological features of childhood RAP have examined a broad range of factors, including life stress, psychological state (anxiety and depression), attention to pain, coping, and parental responses. Due to space limitations, we can only provide a brief summary of this growing literature. For more detailed information, please refer to excellent reviews written by Compas and Boyer (2001), Scharff (1997), and Walker (1999b).

As a whole, investigations of the role of life stress reveal that children with RAP do not experience significantly more major life stressors than healthy children (McGrath, Goodman, Firestone, Shipman, & Peters, 1983; Wasserman, Whitington, & Rivara, 1988), nor do they experience more major stressors than children who have organic abdominal pain (Walker, Garber, & Greene, 1993; Walker & Greene, 1991a). Research on daily life events, however, suggests that daily stress, including events related to family illness, may have a more important role than major stressors in precipitating episodes of abdominal pain. For example, Walker, Garber, Smith, Van Slyke, and Lewis Claar (2001) found that the relation between daily stressors and somatic symptoms was greater for children with RAP than for well children. For more than a third of children with RAP, the relation between stressors and symptoms exceeded a Pearson correlation of .50.

Investigations of anxiety reveal that children with RAP score significantly higher on measures of anxiety than control group children (Campo et al., 2004; Hodges, Kline, Barbero, & Woodruff, 1985). The results of comparisons between children with RAP and children with organic abdominal pain, however, have been inconsistent (Walker et al., 1993; Walker & Greene, 1989). These findings suggest that while anxiety-related symptoms are associated with RAP, they may be the result rather than the cause of pain in at least some children (Walker & Greene, 1989). Interestingly, Dorn et al. (2003) reported that children with RAP and a group with anxiety disorders exhibited psychological symptoms and physiological findings that, in general, had more shared similarities than either group with a physically and psychiatrically healthy control group.

Studies that have examined depressive symptoms have not found consistent differences between children with RAP and control group children (Campo et al., 2004; Hodges, Kline, Barbero, & et al., 1985; McGrath et al., 1983; Raymer, Weininger, & Hamilton, 1984; Walker & Greene, 1989). Depression does not appear to be prevalent in children with RAP, albeit familial depression may play a role in the development of children's abdominal pain (Hodges, Kline, Barbero, & Flanery, 1985). As with anxiety, depressive symptoms in children with RAP may be secondary to underlying chronic pain as opposed to primary in nature (Raymer et al., 1984).

Children with RAP have also been hypothesized to display an attentional bias toward pain stimuli (Compas & Boyer, 2001; Zeltzer Bursch, & Walco, 1997). This bias may increase their focus on environmental pain cues and sensations of pain, increasing their anxiety and fear, which, in turn, exacerbates the pain. Biases in attention have been implicated in the etiology of children's emotional and behavior disorders (e.g., Vasey et al., 1995; Vasey, El-Hag, & Daleiden, 1996) and may also play a role in the development and maintenance of RAP. Consistent with this hypothesis, Thomsen, Compas, Stanger, and Solletti (2000) reported that problems in attentional focus were associated with increased physical symptoms in children with RAP.

As far as coping, existing studies have found that accommodative or secondary control engagement coping (e.g., distraction, acceptance, positive thinking, cognitive restructuring) proves helpful and is related to less pain in children with RAP (Thomsen et al., 2002; Walker, Smith, Garber, & Van Slyke, 1997). Passive or disengagement coping strategies (e.g., denial, cognitive avoidance, behavioral avoidance, wishful thinking), on the other hand, have been associated with increased levels of pain. The results regarding active or primary control coping strategies (e.g., problem solving, emotional expression, emotional modulation, decision making) have been inconsistent. Walker et at. (1997) reported that active coping was related to increased pain, but Thomsen et al. (2000) found no relation between active coping and pain.

Finally, the ways in which parents react or respond to their children's pain may also have an important role in the development and course of RAP. Specifically, positive consequences (e.g., excusing the child from having to do the dishes, allowing the child to stay home from school) may serve to reinforce and maintain pain behaviors and associated functional disability. For example, Walker and Zeman (1992) found that parents encourage children to adopt the sick role for gastrointestinal symptoms (defined as a "stomachache, upset stomach, or abdominal pain) more than for cold symptoms. Children with RAP, compared to well children, reported that their parents more frequently responded to symptom complaints with increased attention and special privileges (Walker et al., 1993).

CLINICAL EVALUATION

Medical Evaluation

Initial medical evaluation of RAP includes a history and thorough physical examination. Limited laboratory screening may include a complete blood count and erythrocyte sedimentation rate, stool studies, and breath hydrogen testing. The goal of this evaluation is to rule out serious, life-threatening physical causes for abdominal pain (Frazer & Rappaport, 1999; Mahajan & Wyllie, 1999).

Psychological Assessment

The psychological assessment, particularly the pain history, is helpful for establishing the diagnosis of RAP and distinguishing among its particular subtypes. Assessment data that shed light on the behavioral processes that maintain a child's symptoms are important for treatment-planning purposes. The format of the psychological assessment of RAP follows from the biopsychosocial model and is highly consistent with the approach utilized in assessment of other recurrent pains, such as headache or chest pain. Attention is given to all psychological and social factors felt to influence the child's pain and functional status, including descriptions of the child's behaviors when experiencing pain, associated functional limitations, and reinforcing consequences maintaining pain behavior (Masek, Russo, & Varni, 1984). For example, an adolescent with RAP may rest or sleep when in pain and miss a considerable amount of school as a result. The adolescent's pain behavior persists because it allows the child to avoid difficult school assignments and stressful social situations. Other factors routinely assessed include the child's mental status, social history (family constellation, school performance, behavioral/social developmental status), medical history (out-of-the-ordinary chronic illness, abnormal developmental milestones) and previous psychological treatment. Table 6.1 presents an outline of areas we typically assess during these interviews.

A variety of questionnaires and rating scales are available for behavioral assessment of RAP. For example, the Varni-Thompson Pediatric Pain Questionnaire (PPQ: Varni, Thompson, & Hanson, 1987) and the Children's Comprehensive Pain Questionnaire (CCPQ: McGrath, 1990) are examples of comprehensive pain assessment tools that can be utilized in assessment of RAP. These measures rely on open-ended items, rating scales, and visual analog scales to evaluate multiple components of a child's pain. Initial studies of the PPQ suggest good convergent validity (Gragg et al., 1996; Varni et al., 1987), stability over time, and sensitivity to changes in physical status and functional ability (Gragg et al., 1996). Studies of the CCPQ suggest that it is also a valid and reliable pain assessment measure (McGrath, 1990). Measures such as the Child Behavior Checklist (CBCL: Achenbach, 1991) and Behavior Assessment System for Children (BASC: Reynolds & Kamphaus, 1998) can be useful for screening and evaluating emotional/behavioral difficulties associated with the child's abdominal pain. The CBCL and BASC are widely used and well-researched rating scales for assessing a broad range of children's emotional/behavior problems.

Over the past several years, a number of questionnaires and checklists have been developed specifically for the purpose of assessing RAP and associated factors. Most of these were developed for research investigations but have

TABLE 6.1. Outline of Clinical Interviews for Assessing Childhood RAP

Brief Meeting with Patient and Parents
Explanation of role of psychologist/behavior therapist
Qualitative description of pain
Onset
Course
Pain parameters (i.e., location, frequency, duration, intensity)
Temporal variations
Situational variations
Other factors that affect pain
Current coping strategies
Previous interventions and outcome (medical, psychological/behavioral, other)

Semistructured Interview with Patient
Impact on daily functioning (school, peer activities, sports/extracurricular activities)
Parental/familial and peer responses
Secondary gain
Academic functioning (grades, learning/behavior problems, special education, prior testing, other school stressors)
Peer relations (friendships, conflict, isolation/withdrawal)
Family (constellation, functioning, problems at home)
Emotional concerns
Life stressors (major life events, daily hassles)
Perceptions of pain (distress level, importance of improvement, perceptions of cause and control)

Semistructured Interview with Parents
Impact on daily functioning (school, peer activities, sports/extracurricular activities)
Parental/familial and peer responses
Secondary gain
Medical/developmental history (out-of-the-ordinary chronic illness, abnormal developmental milestones)
Family medical history
Academic functioning (grades, learning/behavior problems, special education, prior testing, other school stressors)
Peer relations (friendships, conflict, isolation/withdrawal)
Family (constellation, functioning, problems at home, impact of child's pain)
Emotional concerns
Life stressors (major life events, daily hassles)

Behavioral Observations
Congruity between verbal reports of pain and pain behaviors
Familial response to pain behaviors during interviews
Familial response to past medical professionals and prior interventions
General observations of child and family behaviors

clinical utility as well. As components of a comprehensive evaluation of RAP, these measures provide additional sources of data for understanding and treating a child's pain. In our practice, we use these objective measures to supplement information gathered from our interviews with the patient and parents. Refer to Table 6.2 for a list of the measures that we have found helpful.

TABLE 6.2. Questionnaires and Checklists for Assessing Childhood RAP and Associated Factors

---

Symptom-Based Criteria for Childhood Functional Gastrointestinal Disorders
Pediatric Functional Gastrointestinal Disorders Diagnostic Questionnaire
(Schwankovsky & Hyman, 1999)
Questionnaire on Gastrointestinal Symptoms for Children and Adolescents
(Walker, Caplan-Dover, & Rasquin-Weber, 2000)

Abdominal Pain (Frequency, Duration, and Intensity)
Abdominal Pain Index (Walker, Smith, Garber, & Van Slyke, 1997)

Functional Disability
Functional Disability Inventory (Walker & Greene, 1991b)

Coping
Pain Response Inventory (Walker et al., 1997)
Responses to Stress Inventory (Connor-Smith et al., 2000)

Parental Responses to Children=s Pain
Illness Behavior Encouragement Scales (Walker & Zeman, 1992)
Illness Behavior Encouragement Scales—Revised (Van Slyke, 2000)

Finally, a pain diary (see Figure 6.3) provides a method of ongoing behavioral assessment, including pain severity and duration, medication use, and any antecedent events and consequences. The diary that we typically utilize requires entries for each abdominal pain episode and is helpful for establishing the frequency and pattern of a child's pains (Masek, Russo, & Varni, 1984). An alternative for children who have continuous pain is to rate the intensity of their pain at several consistent times on a daily basis (e.g., 7:00 AM, 3:30 PM, 7:30 PM) (Turner, Woolford, & Sanders, 1993). We often request that families begin diaries prior to the initial evaluation and continue to complete them until the conclusion of treatment.

TREATMENT AVENUES

Medical Management

Standard pediatric care for RAP typically consists of reassurance that there is no serious organic disease and general advice about learning to manage pain. When accepted, this reassurance concludes the search for a physical cause and allows the child and family to move into the stage of learning to cope. Although this is important and can be sufficient for some children, medication and psychological therapies are often necessary.

In some cases, symptom-based pharmacological therapies are helpful. For example, tricyclic antidepressants such as desipramine and amitriptyline may be used to target the child's visceral pain. Anticholinergic medications

PAIN RECORD

NAME _____

Hospital
THE CLEVELAND CLINIC

Day of Week	Date Year	Time* Very Important	INTENSITY** CIRCLE ONE	MEDICINES TAKEN? (Type & Amount)	CLASSES OF ACTIVITIES MISSED? (Which ones)	WHAT HAPPENED BEFORE?	WHAT HAPPENED AFTER?
		Start: ___ Stop: ___	Mild Moderate Severe Very Severe				
		Start: ___ Stop: ___	Mild Moderate Severe Very Severe				
		Start: ___ Stop: ___	Mild Moderate Severe Very Severe				
		Start: ___ Stop: ___	Mild Moderate Severe Very Severe				
		Start: ___ Stop: ___	Mild Moderate Severe Very Severe				
		Start: ___ Stop: ___	Mild Moderate Severe Very Severe				
		Start: ___ Stop: ___	Mild Moderate Severe Very Severe				
		Start: ___ Stop: ___	Mild Moderate Severe Very Severe				
		Start: ___ Stop: ___	Mild Moderate Severe Very Severe				
		Start: ___ Stop: ___	Mild Moderate Severe Very Severe				

**Intensity: MILD = You know the pain is there, but it doesn't bother you much. MODERATE = The pain does bother you but can still do things. SEVERE = The pain bothers you a lot, you can't do very much. VERY SEVERE = You can't do anything but rest.

FIGURE 6.3. Pain Record Diary

such as dicyclomine and hyoscyamine have been used for their antispasmodic properties. In those with constipation, targeted therapies (e.g., laxatives, stool softeners) may be a helpful adjunct.

Psychological Treatment

Much of the existing literature on psychological treatments for RAP was summarized in an excellent article by Janicke and Finney (1999). They reviewed the treatment literature available prior to February 1, 1998, and identified nine studies examining three distinctive treatment approaches, including operant procedures (Miller & Kratochwill, 1979; Sank & Biglan, 1974), fiber treatments (Christensen, 1986; Edwards, Finney, & Bonner, 1991; Feldman, McGrath, Hodgson, Ritter, & Shipman, 1985), and cognitive-behavioral procedures (Finney, Lemanek, Cataldo, Katz, & Fuqua, 1989; Linton, 1986; Sanders et al., 1989; Sanders, Shepherd, Cleghorn, & Woolford, 1994). Of note, all patients enrolled in these studies had functional or nonorganic abdominal pain. The extent of medical evaluation that they received was not specified, nor was their medication status certain. Guidelines formulated by the Task Force on Promotion and Dissemination of Psychological Procedures were used to categorize treatments as either well established, probably efficacious, or promising (Chambless et al., 1996). According to these criteria, cognitive-behavioral procedures emerged as a probably efficacious treatment. Fiber treatment for RAP with constipation emerged as a promising intervention. Operant procedures did not meet the most lenient category of empirically supported treatments, and no treatment approach met the criteria for a well-established intervention. Since the publication of Janicke and Finney's article, several other treatment studies have been published. The results of a randomized controlled trail of cognitive-behavioral family treatment (Robins, Smith, Glutting, & Bishop, 2005) add support to the effectiveness of cognitive-behavioral intervention in reducing the sensory aspects of RAP. Other new studies examining biofeedback and self-hypnosis are reviewed later in this chapter.

Cognitive-Behavioral Family Intervention
(Sanders and Colleagues)

One particularly promising psychological treatment is the cognitive-behavioral family intervention by Sanders and his colleagues (Sanders et al., 1989, 1994), which consists of three components delivered in six 50-minute sessions: explanation of RAP and rationale for pain management procedures, contingency management training for parents, and self-management training for children. Among the areas covered in parent training are discriminating between sick and well behaviors, reinforcing well behavior through contingent social attention and token reinforcement, responding to verbal pain complaints by prompting competing behavior or distracting activities, and ignoring nonverbal pain behaviors. As far as self-management, children are taught skills like progressive muscle relaxation, isometric relaxation, imagery, and coping statements. A therapist's manual (Sanders, Patel, & Woolford, 1993) presents a session-by-session outline of treatment strategies. Pain management manuals for children (Turner, Woolford, & Sanders, 1993) and their parents (Turner & Sanders, 1993) are provided to supplement the material covered in each treatment session.

Two studies have evaluated this particular treatment (Sanders et al., 1989, 1994). In their initial study, Sanders et al. (1989) assigned 16 children with RAP to a treatment or wait-list control group. They found that both the treatment group and the control group reduced their levels of pain. However, the treatment group improved quicker, the effects generalized to the school setting, and a larger proportion of subjects were completely pain free by 3-month follow-up (87.5% vs. 37.5%). There was no evidence for any negative effects of treatment. In a second study, Sanders et al. (1994) randomly allocated 44 7- to 14-year-old children to either the cognitive-behavioral family intervention or standard pediatric care (reassurance and general advice). Both treatment conditions resulted in significant improvements on measures of pain intensity and pain behavior. However, the treatment group had a higher rate of complete elimination of pain, lower levels of relapse at 6- and 12-month follow-up, and lower levels of interference with their activities as a result of pain. Parents reported a higher level of satisfaction with the treatment than children receiving standard pediatric care.

Multicomponent Targeted Therapy (Finney and Colleagues)

Though not a standardized treatment protocol, the multicomponent targeted therapy utilized by Finney and his colleagues (Edwards et al., 1991; Finney et al., 1989) also warrants attention. This therapy is based on a behavioral medicine approach that considers biological and behavioral etiologies and treatment factors. The therapy includes procedures designed to teach children to monitor the frequency and intensity of pain episodes, determine situations in which pain occurs frequently, reduce parental attention for recurrent pain, teach a relaxation procedure as a coping response, increase dietary fiber intake, and increase functional activities. Specific procedures include self-monitoring, limited reinforcement of illness behavior, relaxation training, dietary food supplementation, and participation in routine activities. Intervention is tailored for each patient based on behavioral concerns and symptoms identified during the assessment process. Thus, one child may receive only one or a few procedures, while another child receives all five procedures. For example, a child who does not miss school due to RAP and only infrequently discusses pain episodes with parents would not receive the participation in routine activities and limited reinforcement procedures. The therapy is brief in nature, with the number of therapy visits in controlled investigations ranging from one to six visits over a period of 1 to 6 months. Although there is obviously overlap between the techniques employed by Sanders and colleagues and those utilized by Finney et al., the multicomponent targeted approach acknowledges the uniqueness of each case and facilitates matching of treatment components with target areas delineated during the assessment.

Two studies have evaluated the multicomponent targeted therapy approach. In an initial evaluation, Finney et al. (1989) treated 16 children with RAP who were referred to a primary care-based pediatric psychology service. After treatment, improvement or resolution of pain symptoms was reported for 13 (81%) children, and school absences were significantly decreased. Medical care utilization significantly decreased after treatment, whereas a comparison group of untreated children with RAP showed no change in medical care visits over time. In a second investigation, Edwards et al. (1991) assigned 11 children to dietary fiber or relaxation treatments based upon whether they presented with symptoms of constipation. Use of fiber was found to be associated with improvement in patients with symptoms of constipation. Relaxation treatment achieved only minimal success for children without constipation.

Alternative Treatments

Despite the growing evidence base for conventional interventions, interest in alternative treatments for RAP is expanding. Much of this interest stems from the fact that not all children with RAP benefit from conventional treatments. Unfortunately, the empirical support for alternative treatments lags behind the interest level. In our literature search, we identified papers on the following alternative intervention strategies: biofeedback therapy, hypnotherapy, acupuncture, peppermint oil, and folk remedies. Some of the studies included children as well as adult participants. These studies were not exclusively limited to children with pain of a functional nature, and some included children with organic pain as well. Because of the increased interest in alternatives, familiarity with this literature is important. As more is learned about the efficacy and safety of certain alternative treatments for RAP, integration of these strategies and conventional treatments are expected to grow.

Various types of biofeedback therapy have been used to treat RAP. Electrocardiogram and pneumograph biofeedback provide the patient and the practitioner with valuable information for effective treatment of RAP. Electrocardiogram (ECG) biofeedback devices with the capability to separate cardiac rhythms into separate spectral bands are able to calculate the patient's vagal tone, an indicator of their autonomic nervous system's ability to achieve and maintain homeostasis. By watching the display of moment-to-moment psychological activity with the patient, the practitioner can coach the patient in resonant frequency training by instructing him or her to increase activity in the low frequency range and decrease activity in the very low and high frequency ranges. This method of focusing on the "peak" of activity in the low frequency range is an efficient method of familiarizing the patient with his or her own unique physiological response. The practitioner and patient can also validate the intervention by monitoring session-to-session improvements and comparing them to changes in the patient's pain frequency or severity.

Pneumograph (PNG) biofeedback monitors respiratory activity to facilitate training in abdominal breathing, a particularly helpful treatment for RAP. With strain gauges around both the chest and abdomen, the patient learns to decrease chest movement and increase abdominal movement. The practitioner also explains the effects of shallow breathing and demonstrates with a capnometer, when available. With this guidance, the patient learns to breathe fully, slowly, and evenly, utilizing the diaphragm muscle.

Additionally, electrodermograph (EDG) biofeedback, consisting of skin conductance/resistance, can be used for training the patient to reduce worry and anxiety, and thermal biofeedback, measuring peripheral skin temperature, can be used to vasodilate and enhance blood flow. Electromyography (EMG) can be used to train the patient in muscle relaxation, if indicated. Each of these types of biofeedback provides immediate feedback, which assists the learning process as well as the patient's sense of control and understanding of personal physiology.

In a study examining biofeedback as one component of a behavioral treatment protocol for RAP, Humphreys and Gervitz (2000) compared four different treatment protocols using a pretest-posttest control group design. Participants in the research were 64 children and adolescents with RAP. They were randomly assigned into four groups: (1) fiber-only comparison group; (2) fiber and skin temperature biofeedback; (3) fiber, skin temperature biofeedback, and cognitive-behavioral procedures; and (4) fiber, skin temperature biofeedback, cognitive-behavioral procedures, and contingency management training for parents. The results revealed that all groups showed improvement in self-reported pain. The active treatment groups, however, showed significantly more improvement than the fiber-only comparison group. Because the addition of cognitive-behavioral parent support components did not seem to increase treatment effectiveness, the authors concluded that increased fiber with biofeedback-assisted low arousal was effective and efficient as a treatment modality for RAP.

As for hypnotherapy, Anbar (2001) published a case series to demonstrate the utility of self-hypnosis for the treatment of childhood functional abdominal pain. In four of five patients, abdominal pain resolved within 3 weeks of a single session of self-hypnosis instruction. Sokel, Devane, and Bentovim (1991) reported that all 6 of their RAP patients were able to use self-hypnosis to reduce or remove pain so that they were able to resume normal activities within a mean period of 17.6 days. Browne (1997) reported that 7 children with RAP were treated with brief hypnotherapy and subsequently rated at follow-up as improved. In another study, Ball, Shapiro, Monheim, and Weydert (2003) found that children with long-standing RAP that was refractory to conventional therapy had a decrease in their complaints of abdominal pain during and following relaxation and mental imagery, the two primary components of pediatric hypnotherapy. Though encouraging, these studies are limited by the absence of prospective-controlled designs and inconsistent use of objective measures of improvement.

Two acupuncture studies were identified. Yanhua and Sumei (2000) reported on the treatment of 86 cases of epigastric and abdominal pain by scalp acupuncture. Significant improvement resulted from the insertion of just a few needles. Xiaoma (1988) described electroimpulse acupuncture treatment of 110 cases were clinically cured with disappearance of symptoms and signs. These studies had mixed age samples and, like the hypnotherapy studies, were not prospective controlled investigations. The latter study assessed children with presumably organic pain, and the extent to which its findings can be generalized to functional abdominal pain is uncertain.

In a randomized, double-blind controlled study (Kline, Kline, DiPalma, & Barbero, 2001), 42 children with irritable bowel syndrome (a subtype of RAP) were given pH-dependent, enteric-coated peppermint oil capsules or placebo. After 2 weeks, 75% of those receiving peppermint oil had reduced severity of pain associated with IBS.

Finally, a study of folk remedies for a Hispanic population (Risser & Mazur, 1995) found that tea (chamomile, cinnamon, honey, and lemon) was commonly used to treat childhood abdominal pain. Participants were 51 Hispanic caregivers, mostly mothers, attending a primary care facility serving a primarily Hispanic population. The authors failed to specify whether the children's pain was functional or organically caused. No outcome data were reported.

PRACTICE ISSUES AND RECOMMENDATIONS

In our clinical practice, we utilize a cognitive-behavioral systems approach that integrates various aspects of the treatments developed by Sanders and colleagues (Sanders et al., 1989, 1994) and Finney and colleagues (Edwards et al., 1991; Finney et al., 1989). Our approach is consistent with other behavioral approaches to the management of chronic pain in children (Masek, Russo, & Varni, 1984). Like Sanders and colleagues, our treatment consists of three components: explanation of RAP and rationale for cognitive-behavioral pain management training, pain behavior management training for parents, and self-regulation training for children. Our aims are to reduce pain perception and behavioral distress, increase functional behaviors, and modify social, familial, and life factors that precipitate and maintain pain. Similar to Finney and colleagues, the content and nature of the parent- and child-skills training is tailored for each patient (see appendix A.)

Our experience is that optimal treatment of RAP follows from a treatment plan that most closely matches the child's presentation (Edwards et al., 1991; Finney et al., 1989). For example, while the addition of a parental support component may not enhance outcome for all subtypes of RAP (Humphreys & Gervitz, 2000), parental support can be immensely beneficial when there is evidence of inadvertent parental reinforcement of pain behavior. A combined treatment comprised of multiple components, such as the Sanders et al. intervention, may, in fact, be the optimal intervention for RAP children whose presentation warrants a comprehensive approach. A simpler treatment, possibly emphasizing increased fiber or biofeedback alone, may be sufficient for RAP associated with one particular problem or deficit. Family resources should also be considered. For example, while the complexity of some cases may suggest the need for comprehensive treatment, the demands of such a program may make these treatments difficult to implement with all families.

Reassurance and Education

Reassurance that there is no serious organic disease and education about RAP are essential first steps in the treatment process. Acknowledgment that the child's pain is real but not life threatening is critical (Hyman, 1999). When understood and accepted, this reassurance prompts the child and family to end their search for a physical cause for the pain and encourages them to move into the next stage of learning to cope or manage. Presentation of a biopsychosocial model in which a child's RAP is presumed to be a function of multiple interacting factors, including psychological and social influences (Drossman, 2000), sets the stage for behavioral intervention. Crushell et al. (2003) found that only 7% of parents of children with ongoing abdominal pain believed that there was a psychological cause for their child's pain, whereas 78% of the children who no longer had pain believed that the cause was attributable to psychological factors. They concluded that the acceptance by parents of a biopsychosocial model of illness is important for the resolution of childhood RAP.

An important aspect of the educational process is discussion of treatment goals. We emphasize that the goals of behavioral treatment are to help children learn to manage their pain independently and to promote normal daily activity despite the pain. We note that the practice and use of the coping strategies taught may not totally eliminate pain but may result in shorter and less severe pain episodes. In our experience, children and parents who have appropriate expectations tend to be more compliant and satisfied with treatment.

Parent Management Training

It is essential to teach parents to discriminate between sick role and well behaviors and avoid modeling sick behaviors. Contingency management training assists parents in reinforcing practice and use of pain management strategies and promoting functional behaviors in the face of pain. We instruct parents to encourage normal patterns of daily activity and discourage pain and related problem behaviors (Masek, Russo, & Varni, 1984). Contingent social attention and token reinforcement in the form of a happy faces or points chart are both effective strategies.

Self-Regulation Training for Children

No particular pain management strategy will be effective for all children across all pain episodes. As such, we teach children a variety of pain management or self-regulation strategies, explaining that the more coping skills children have, the more effective they will be. Our aim is to help children learn to manage their pain independently or, as we state to them, "learn to be the boss of their body." Among the strategies typically taught are relaxation/mental imagery, cognitive coping, diaphragmatic breathing, autogenics, and progressive muscle relaxation. The training process is accomplished through a combination of verbal and written instructions, within-session demonstrations and practice techniques, and specific weekly homework tasks. Children are encouraged to practice and apply new strategies, with an eye on identifying those techniques that they find most helpful.

Increasing Functional Behaviors

Another issue for consideration in the treatment of RAP is the daily functional status of the child. In some children, RAP becomes disabling, leading to poor school attendance, limited extracurricular activities, and other impairments in daily functioning. Bursch and colleagues (Bursch, 1999; Bursch, Walco, & Zeltzer, 1998) coined the term *Pain Associated Disability Syndrome* (PADS) to describe the severe manifestation of this clinical phenomenon. PADS is defined as a downward spiral of increasing pain-associated disability, lasting at least 3 months, for which symptom-focused strategies have not led to an acceptable resolution. Although elimination of the pain is the most desired treatment outcome, this goal may not be realistic for all children with RAP. Increased focus on the child's functional status acknowledges this possibility, shifting attention to the child's quality of life despite the presence of symptoms. In our experience, this shift requires focused attention on the child's functional status and the implementation of treatment components that specifically target increased daily activity. For example, Benore, Wertalik, Beck, and Slifer (2004) reported that shifting a family's focus from pain to adaptive functioning resulted in less termination of pleasurable activities, fewer school absences, and longer outings.

Modifying Social, Familial, and Life Contributors

Though the contributions of life stress are not explicitly addressed in existing treatment protocols, they may warrant considerable attention in clinical practice. Identification of life stressors that trigger pain episodes and recognition of their impact on the child's ability to cope are important. From session to session, we monitor the relation between life stress and episodes of abdominal pain via the pain diary. Over the course of treatment, the stressors that trigger pain often receive increased attention. For some children, we have found that assistance in coping with these stressors is as or more critical than formal pain management training.

Finally, it not uncommon for the child with RAP to have parents or other family members who also have recurrent pains or other somatic complaints. Walker and Greene (1989) reported that anxiety, depression, and somatization were greater in mothers of children with RAP than mothers of well children. Wasserman et al. (1988) found a higher incidence of current and prior painful gastrointestinal disorders among family members of children with RAP than among family members of well children. The presence of family members with recurrent pains and associated functional disability complicates the process of treating RAP. Familial modeling and support of maladaptive pain behaviors may diminish the child's motivation to learn to manage recurring abdominal pain. In such cases, behavioral treatment may not be sufficient, and more intensive family therapy focused on the functions served by the pain and the processes maintaining it may be warranted.

APPENDIX A

Sample Treatment Protocol

Initial Treatment Session

1. Review pain diary (look for temporal patterns, psychosocial stressors, and physical precipitants.)
2. Reassurance and education:
   - Reassure that there is no serious organic disease and educate about RAP.
   - Provide biopsychosocial conceptualization, with attention to social learning factors (e.g., inadvertent reinforcement of pain behavior).
   - Introduce the concept of self-management.
   - Establish appropriate expectations, including improvement of functional status.
3. Self-regulation skills training:
   - Use clinical judgment to help patients select a starting method (i.e., progressive muscle relaxation, relaxation via letting go, imagery, or autogenics).
   - A combination of methods, such as progressive muscle and an imagery technique, is often used.

- Tape record the entire sequence as you instruct the patient for the first time in the office. The tape should be about 10 minutes long.
- Establish a home practice schedule (once per day as a firm commitment is recommended, with a second optional practice per day).

4. Bring parents in at the end, and praise patient for his or her initial efforts. Review practice requirement with parents. Continue pain diary. Schedule next visit in 1 to 2 weeks.

Sessions 2–4

1. Subsequent treatment sessions are typically scheduled 1 to 2 weeks apart.
2. Review pain data, relaxation tape practice, and other clinical information.
3. Implement behavioral procedures to improve compliance with relaxation practice, if indicated.
4. Introduce pain behavior management guidelines for parents (see Table 6.3). Tailor guidelines to match patient's presentation and emphasize adaptive functioning.
5. Continue self-regulation skills training. During session three or four, tape record another relaxation procedure on the other side and have patients shift home practice to the new procedure. The second side of the tape should be shorter (around 6 to 7 minutes) and focus more on cue-controlled relaxation (i.e., diaphragmatic breathing coupled with a word or special image).

TABLE 6.3. Pain Management Guidelines for Parents

Encourage Normal Activity
Express frequent approval for maintaining activity patterns.
Encourage child to stay calm and practice relaxation where feasible.
Advocate daily school attendance or stay in school as the norm.

Discourage Pain Behavior
Ignore excessive complaining, pain gestures, and request for special treatment and assistance. Instruct others to do the same if necessary.
Dispense medications for symptomatic relief according to directions and follow recommended time sequence.
Evaluate whether the consequence of the pain behavior is to avoid or escape from an activity or situation. If so, consider maintaining things as they are *or* introduce an alternative (e.g., bed rest) that has little appeal to child.
Avoid questioning about presence of pain or status of pain.

Source: Masek, Russo, & Varni (1984).

Subsequent Treatment Sessions

6. Review pain behavior management guidelines for parents. Revise as necessary. If indicated, implement formal reward/reinforcement program.
7. Implement cognitive-behavioral procedures for stress management/ problem solving, as indicated. Self-statement modification and thought-stopping help the patient shut down unhelpful thoughts about pain/self and replace them with healthful, positive messages. Problem-solving strategies can be taught as a way of coping with pain-related stressors.
8. Assist the patient and family in modifying social/familial contributors to pain.
9. Discuss high-risk situations and introduce notion of relapse prevention. Use role plays and problem solving to prepare the child and parents for difficult situations that may arise in relation to pain management.
10. Treatment is typically 4 to 8 sessions in duration.

Follow-Up

1. Schedule the first follow-up appointment 4 to 6 weeks after the last treatment session. Schedule additional follow-ups at 3 to 6 months.

REFERENCES

Achenbach, T. M. (1991). *Manual of the Child Behavior Checklist/4-18 and 1991 Profile* (CBCL). Burlington, VT: University of Vermont. University Associates of Psychiatry.

Anbar, R. D. (2001). Self-hypnosis for the treatment of functional abdominal pain in childhood. *Clinical Pediatrics, 40,* 447–451.

Apley, J. (1959). *The child with abdominal pain.* London: Blackwell.

Apley, J. (1975). *The child with abdominal pains* (2nd ed.). London: Blackwell.

Apley, J., & Hale, B. (1973). Children with recurrent abdominal pain: How do they grow up? *British Medical Journal, 7,* 7–9.

Apley, J., & Naish, N. (1958). Recurrent abdominal pain: A field survey of 1,000 school children. *Archives of Diseases of Childhood, 33,* 165–170.

Ball, T. M., Shapiro, D. E., Monheim, C. J., & Weydert, J. A. (2003). A pilot study of the use of guided imagery for the treatment of abdominal pain in children. *Clinical Pediatrics, 42,* 527–532.

Benore, E., Wertalik, G., Beck, M., & Slifer, K. (2004). *Shifting the focus from pain: The effect of child and family therapy targeting adaptive functioning in managing recurrent pain.* Paper presented at the National Conference on Child Health Psychology, Charleston, SC.

Campo, J. V., Ehmann, M., Altman, S., Lucas, A., Birmaher, B., DiLorenzo, C., Iyengar, S., & Brent, D. A. (2004). Recurrent abdominal pain, anxiety, and depression in primary care. *Pediatrics, 113,* 817–824.

Chambless, D., Sanderson, W. C., Shoham, V., Johnson, S. B., Pope, K. S., Crits-Cristoph, P. et al. (1996). An update on empirically validated therapies. *Clinical Psychologist, 49,* 5–18.

Christensen, M. F. (1986). Recurrent abdominal pain and dietary fiber. *American Journal of Diseases in Children, 140*, 738–739.k

Christensen, M. F., & Mortensen, O. (1975). Long-term prognosis in children with recurrent abdominal pain. *Archives of Diseases of Childhood, 50*, 110–115.

Compas, B. E., & Boyer, M. C. (2001). Coping and attention: Implications for child health and pediatric conditions. *Journal of Developmental and Behavioral Pediatrics, 22*, 323–333.

Crushell, E., Rowland, M., Doherty, M., Gormally, S., Harty, S., Bourke, B. et al. (2003). Importance of parental conceptual model of illness in severe recurrent abdominal pain. *Pediatrics, 112*, 1368–1372.

Dorn, L. D., Campo, J. C., Thato, S., Dahl, R. E., Lewin, D., Chandra, R. et al. (2003). Psychological comorbidity and stress reactivity in childrena and adolescents with recurrent abdominal pain and anxiety disorders. *Journal of the American Academy of Child and Adolescent Psychiatry, 42*, 66–75.

Drossman, D. A. (2000). The functional gastrointestinal disorders and the Rome II process. In D. A. Drossman, E. Corazziari, N. J. Talley, W. G. Thompson, W. E. Whitehead (Eds.), *Rome II: The functional gastrointestinal disorders* (pp. 1–29). Lawrence, KS: Allen Press.

Duarte, M. A., Goulart, E. M., & Penna, F. J. (2000). Pressure pain threshold in children with recurrent abdominal pain. *Journal of Pediatric Gastroenterology and Nutrition, 31*, 280–285.

Edwards, M. C., Finney, J. W., & Bonner, M. (1991). Matching treatment with recurrent abdominal pain symptoms: An evaluation of dietary fiber and relaxation treatments. *Behavior Therapy, 20*, 283–291.

El-Matary, W., Spray, C., & Sandu, B. (2004). Irritable bowel syndrome: The commonest cause of recurrent abdominal pain in children. *European Journal of Pediatrics, 163*, 584–588.

Feldman, W., McGrath, P., Hodgeson, C., Ritter, H., & Shipman, R.T. (1985). The use of dietary fiber in the management of simple, childhood, idiopathic, recurrent, abdominal pain. *Archives of Diseases of Childhood, 139*, 1216–1218.

Finney, J. W., Lemanek, K. L., Cataldo, M. F., Katz, H. P., & Fuqua, R. W. (1989). Pediatric psychology in primary health care: Brief targeted therapy for recurrent abdominal pain. *Behavior Therapy, 20*, 283–291.

Frazer, C. H., & Rappaport, L. A. (1999). Recurrent pains. In M. D. Levine, W. B. Carey, & A. C. Crocker (Eds.), *Developmental-behavioral pediatrics* (pp. 357–364). Philadelphia: W. B. Saunders.

Hodges, K., Kline, J. J., Barbero, G., & Flanery, R. (1985). Depressive symptoms in children with recurrent abdominal and in their families. *Journal of Pediatrics, 107*, 622–626.

Hodges, K., Kline, J. J., Barbero, G., & Woodruff, C. (1985). Anxiety in children with recurrent abdominal pain and in their parents. *Psychosomatics, 26*, 859–866.

Humphreys, P. A., & Gervitz, R. N. (2000). Treatment of recurrent abdominal pain: Components analysis of four treatment protocols. *Journal of Pediatric Gastroenterology and Nutrition, 31*, 47–51.

Hyams, J. S., Burke, G., Davis, P. M., Rzepsaki, B., & Andrulonis, P. A. (1996). Abdominal pain and irritable bowel syndrome in adolescents: A community-based study. *Journal of Pediatrics, 129*, 220–226.

Janicke, D. M., & Finney, J. W. (1999). Empirically supported treatments in pediatric psychology: Recurrent abdominal pain. *Journal of Pediatric Psychology, 24*, 115–127.

Levine, M. D., & Rappaport, L. A. (1984). Recurrent abdominal pain in school children: The loneliness of the long-distance physician. *Pediatric Clinics of North America, 31*, 969–991.

Linton, S. J. (1986). A case study of the behavioural treatment of chronic stomach pain in a child. *Behaviour Change, 3*, 70–73.

Mahajan, L., & Wyllie, R. (1999). Chronic abdominal pain of childhood and adolescence. In R. Wyllie & J. S. Hyams (Eds.), *Pediatric gastrointestinal disease: Pathophysiology, diagnosis, & management* (pp. 3–13). Philadelphia: W. B. Saunders.

Masek, B. J., Russo, D. C., & Varni, J. W. (1984). Behavioral approaches to the management of chronic pain in children. *Pediatric Clinics of North America, 31*, 1113–1131.

McGrath, P. A. (1990). *Pain in children: Nature, assessment, and treatment.* New York: Guilford.

McGrath, P. J., Goodman, J. T., Firestone, P., Shipman, R., & Peters, S. (1983). Recurrent abdominal pain: A psychogenic disorder? *Archives of Diseases in Childhood, 58,* 888–890.

Miller, A. J., & Kratochwill, T. R. (1979). Reduction of frequent stomach complaints by time out. *Behavior Therapy, 10,* 211–218.

Oster, J. (1972). Recurrent abdominal pain, headache and limb pains in children and adolescents. *Pediatrics, 50,* 429–436.

Rasquin-Weber, A., Hyman P. E., Cucchiara, S., Fleisher, D. R., Hyams, J. S., Milla, P. J., & Staiano, A. (1999). Childhood functional gastrointestinal disorders. *Gut, 45*(Suppl. 2), 1160–1168.

Raymer, D., Weininger, O., & Hamilton, J. R. (1984). Psychological problems in children with abdominal pain. *Lancet, 1,* 439–440.

Reynolds, C. R., & Kamphaus, R. W. (1998). *Behavior assessment system for children: Manual.* Circle Pineas, MN: American Guidance Service.

Robins, P. M., Smith, S. M., Glutting, J. J., & Bishop, C. T. (2005). A randomized controlled trail of a cognitive-behavioral family intervention for pediatric recurrent abdominal pain. *Journal of Pediatric Psychology, 30,* 397–408.

Sanders, M. R., Rebgetz, M., Morrison, M. M., Bor, W., Gordon, A., Dadds, M. R. et al. (1989). Cognitive-behavioral treatment of recurrent nonspecific abdominal pain in children: An analysis of generalization, and maintenance side effects. *Journal of Consulting and Clinical Psychology, 57,* 294–300.

Sanders, M. R., Shepherd, R. W., Cleghorn, G., & Woolford, H. (1994). The treatment of recurrent abdominal pain in children: A controlled comparison of cognitive-behavioral family intervention and standard pediatric care. *Journal of Consulting and Clinical Psychology, 62,* 306–314.

Sank, L. I., & Biglan, A. (1974). Operant treatment of a case of recurrent abdominal pain in a 10-year-old boy. *Behavior Therapy, 5,* 677–681.

Scharff, L. (1997). Recurrent abdominal pain in children: A review of psychological factors and treatment. *Clinical Psychology Review, 17,* 145–166.

Schwankovsky, L., & Hyman, P. E. (1999). Pediatric functional gastrointestinal disorders diagnostic questionnaire. In P. E. Hyman (Ed.), *Pediatric functional gastrointestinal disorders* (pp. A1–A8). New York: Academy Professional Information Services.

Stickler, G. B., & Murphy, D. B. (1979). Recurrent abdominal pain. *American Journal of Diseases in Childhood, 133,* 486–489.

Stordal, K., Nygaard, E. A., & Bentsen, B. S. (2005). Recurrent abdominal pain: A five year follow-up study. *Acta Paediatrica, 94,* 234–236.

Thomsen, A. H., Compas, B. E., Colletti, R. B., Stanger, C., Boyer, M. C., & Konik, B. S. (2002). Parent reports of coping and stress responses in children with recurrent abdominal pain. *Journal of Pediatric Psychology, 27,* 215–226.

Thomsen, A. H., Compas, B. E., Colletti, R. B., & Stanger, C. (2000). *Self-report of coping and stress responses in adolescents with recurrent abdominal pain.* Manuscript submitted for publication.

Varni, J. W., Thompson, K. L., & Hanson, V. (1987). The Varni/Thompson Pediatric pain questionnaire. I. Chronic musculoskeletal pain in juvenile rheumatoid arthritis. *Pain, 28,* 27–38.

Vasey, M. W., Daleiden, E.L., Williams, L. L., & Brown, L. (1995). Biased attention in childhood anxiety disorders: A preliminary study. *Journal of Abnormal Child Psychology, 23,* 267–279.

Vasey M. W., El-Hag, N., & Daleiden, E. L. (1996). Anxiety and the processing of emotionally-threatening stimuli: Dissociative patterns of selective attention among high- and- low-test-anxious children. *Child Development, 67,* 1173–1185.

Von Baeyer, C. L., & Walker, L. S. (1999). Children with recurrent abdominal pain: Issues in the selection and description of research participants. *Journal of Developmental and Behavioral Pediatrics, 20,* 307–313.

Walker, L. S. (1999a). Pathways between recurrent abdominal pain and adult functional gastrointestinal disorders. *Journal of Developmental and Behavioral Pediatrics, 20,* 320–321.

Walker, L. S. (1999b). The evolution of research on recurrent abdominal pain: History, assumptions, and a conceptual model. In P. J. McGrath & G. A. Finley (Eds.), *Chronic and recurrent pain in children and adolescents* (pp. 141–172). Seattle: International Association for the Study of Pain.

Walker, L. S., Caplan-Dover, A., Rasquin-Weber, A. (2000). *Questionnaire on gastrointestinal symptoms for children and adolescents.* Unpublished manuscript.

Walker, L. S., Garber, J., & Greene, J. W. (1993). Psychosocial correlates of recurrent childhood pain: A comparison of pediatric patients with recurrent abdominal pain, organic illness, and psychiatric disorders. *Journal of Abnormal of Psychology, 102*, 248–258.

Walker, L. S., Garber, J., Smith, C. A., Van Slyke, D. A., & Lewis Claar, R. (2001). The relation of daily stressors to somatic and emotional symptoms in children with and without recurrent abdominal pain. *Journal of Consulting and Clinical Psychology, 69*, 85–91.

Walker, L. S., & Green, J. W. (1989). Children with recurrent abdominal pain and their parents: More somatic complaints, anxiety, and depression than other parent groups? *Journal of Pediatric Psychology, 12*, 231–224.

Walker, L. S., & Greene, J. W. (1991a). Negative life events and symptom resolution in pediatric abdominal pain patients. *Journal of Pediatric Psychology, 16*, 341–360.

Walker, L. S., & Greene, J. W. (1991b). The functional disability inventory measuring a neglected dimension of child health status. *Journal of Pediatric Psychology, 16*, 39–58.

Walker, L. S., Smith, C. A., Garber, J., & Van Slyke, D. A. (1997). Development and validation of the Pain Response Inventory for Children. *Psychological Assessment, 9*, 392–405.

Walker, L. S., & Zeman, J. L. (1992). Parental response to child illness behavior. *Journal of Pediatric Psychology, 17*, 49–71.

Wasserman, A. L., Whitington, P. F., & Rivara, F. P. (1988). Psychogenic basis for abdominal pain in children and adolescents. *Journal of the American Academy of Child and Adolescent Psychiatry, 27*, 179–184.

Youseff, N. N., & DiLorenzo, C. (2001). The role of motility in functional abdominal disorders in children. *Pediatric Annals, 30*, 24–30.

Zeltzer, L., Bursch, B., & Walco, G. (1997). Pain responsiveness and chronic pain: A psychobiological perspective. *Journal of Developmental and Behavioral Pediatrics, 18*, 413–422.

Zuckerman, B., Stevenson, J., & Bailey, V. (1986). Stomachaches and headaches in a community sample of preschool children. *Pediatrics, 79*, 677–682.

Irritable Bowel Syndrome

Irritable bowel syndrome (IBS) is a functional gastrointestinal disorder characterized by chronic or recurrent abdominal pain/discomfort, altered bowel function (urgency, altered stool consistency, altered stool frequency, incomplete evacuation), and bloating/distention. These symptoms are felt to stem from the function of the bowels. They are not explained by identifiable structural or biochemical abnormalities. The two most commonly used symptom-based criteria for IBS are the Manning criteria (Manning, Thompson, Heating, & Morris, 1978) and the Rome criteria (Thompson et al., 2000; Thompson et al., 1999). These criteria were originally developed for adults, but have been successfully used with children and adolescents. The Manning criteria were established to differentiate IBS from organic disease in patients attending an outpatient gastroenterology clinic. They have been used for patient selection in epidemiological studies and clinical trials and have served their original purpose well. The Manning criteria include the following: (1) visible abdominal distention, (2) relief of pain with bowel movement, (3) more frequent bowel movements with the onset of pain, (4) loose stools at onset of pain, (5) passage of mucous per rectum, and (6) feeling of incomplete evacuation. The Rome criteria resulted from consensus conferences to define criteria for a broad range of functional gastrointestinal disorders. The most recent version, the Rome II criteria (Rasquin-Weber et al., 1999), have emerged as the gold standard and require that the primary IBS symptoms must be continuous or recurrent for at least 3 months. The abdominal pain or discomfort has two or three features: (1) it is relieved with defecation, (2) associated with a change in frequency of stool, and/or (3) associated with a change in form of stool. No structural or metabolic abnormalities explain the symptoms. According to Rome II criteria, symptoms that cumulatively support the diagnosis of IBS include: abnormal stool frequency (> 3 BMs/day or < 3 BMs/week); abnormal stool form (lumpy/hard or loose/watery stool); abnormal stool passage (straining, urgency, or feeling of incomplete evaluation); passage of mucous; and bloating or feeling of abdominal distention. When appropriate, the Rome II criteria classify IBS as either "diarrhea-predominant" or "constipation-predominant" on the basis of the predominant bowel habit. For some individuals, diarrhea and constipation alternate.

Within the Rome classification scheme, IBS is categorized as one subtype of abdominal pain. Others include functional dyspepsia, functional abdominal pain, abdominal migraine, and aerophagia. Altered bowel function (i.e., diarrhea, constipation) distinguishes IBS from the other abdominal pain disorders. IBS has also been conceptualized as a later stage manifestation of the recurrent nonorganic abdominal pain seen in childhood. For example, Walker and her colleagues (1998) reported that 5 years after their initial evaluation, patients with RAP were more likely than female controls to meet the Manning criteria for IBS. These data suggest that females with a childhood history of RAP may be at particular risk for the development of IBS.

It is important to note that some practitioners use the term IBS loosely to describe any functional abdominal pain, whether or not disordered defecation is present. Though there may be a clinical argument for this practice (i.e., a positive diagnosis of IBS may be more acceptable than that of nonorganic pain), this usage hinders provider and patient communication and potentially affects selection of the most appropriate treatment. Clearly, the more that symptom-based criteria are utilized, the better our understanding and treatment of IBS will be. The majority of the studies cited in this chapter utilized symptom-based criteria. The few pediatric IBS investigations will be emphasized, but both adult and child studies are included.

CAUSES AND CONCEPTUALIZATION

The cause of IBS has not been definitively established. Multiple factors are thought to contribute, including physiological factors, such as abnormal motility (increased or irregular movement of the gut), enhanced visceral sensitivity, intestinal inflammation, and brain physiology, as well as psychosocial factors, such as stress (American Digestive Health Foundation, 2001). As is the case with recurrent abdominal pain (see Chapter 6), the etiology and course of IBS is increasingly conceptualized from a biopsychosocial perspective (Drossman, 1998). The patient's IBS symptoms and daily functioning are presumed to be a function of multiple factors and their interactions along the central nervous system/enteric nervous system or "brain-gut" axis. In people with IBS, the nerve endings in the lining of the bowel are thought to be unusually sensitive, and the nerves that control the muscles of the gut are highly active. Symptoms appear to be the result of increased sensitivity to distension of the gastrointestinal tract by gas or fecal material (normal events) and a tendency for the bowel to be overly reactive to almost anything: eating, stress, emotional arousal, or gaseous distension. Individuals with IBS react to these events by developing more pronounced contractions in the bowel, and these contractions seem to be responsible for the sensations of bloating, discomfort, and urgency.

The role of stress and other psychosocial factors is multifaceted. While psychosocial stressors do not cause IBS, they can clearly exacerbate a patient's gastrointestinal symptoms (Bennett, Tennant, Piesse, Badcock, & Kellow, 1998). Stressors also affect an individual's symptom experience, efforts to cope, and eventual clinical outcome (Drossman, 1999; Gaynes & Drossman, 1999). The symptoms themselves can become a source of stress that impacts daily functioning. Although stressors can affect bowel function in anyone, the effect appears greater in people with IBS. Stress may also impact on the health care utilization of patients with IBS. For example, psychiatric comorbidity is more prevalent among IBS patients who are heavy users of medical services.

The abdominal pain, altered bowel habits, and associated psychological factors all can contribute to a significant negative quality of life impact (Hahn, Yan, & Strassels, 1999). Patients with IBS have rated their quality of life as being lower than both the national norm and patients with type II diabetes (Wells et al., 1997). IBS is the second most common cause of work and school absenteeism, the first being the common cold. It can lead patients to miss work or school or to arrive late or leave early because of an IBS episode. According to a recent survey (IFFGD, 2002), IBS symptoms caused missed leisure activities even more than absenteeism at work or school. Missed leisure activities were reported as occurring among over two thirds of the respondents (68%), with 5% reporting missing such occasions more than 50 times in a 3-month period. For children and adolescents with IBS, missed school, peer activities, and sports/extracurricular activities are not uncommon when symptoms are severe. According to the biopsychosocial model, these problems in daily function directly affect the patient's subsequent symptom experience and coping behavior.

PREVALENCE

Ten to 20% of all adults experience symptoms of IBS. IBS is the most common diagnosis among gastroenterology practices in the United States (Everhart & Renault, 1991) and one of the top ten reasons for primary care visits (PDDA, 1999). The prevalence of IBS is significantly greater in women than in men (ratio 2:1) (Sandler, 1990). Moreover, females are three times more likely than males to seek medical attention (Drossman, Whitehead, & Camilleri, 1997). Interestingly, almost 75% of IBS sufferers do not consult with a physician for their symptoms. Among the 25% of IBS consulters, most see their primary care practitioner for their symptoms. Only a small minority see IBS subspecialists.

IBS is also common in children and adolescents. In a population-based study of 507 middle and high school students from a suburban town in Connecticut (Hyams, Burke, Davis, Rzepski, & Andrulonis, 1996), 6% of middle school students and 14% of high school students reported symptoms consistent with a diagnosis of IBS. The likelihood of seeing a physician was four times greater in those students whose pain affected their activities. In a medical practice-based study (Hyams et al., 1995), IBS-like symptoms were present in the majority of 227 children and adolescents presenting to a pediatric gastroenterology clinic with recurrent abdominal pain. Of the 171 patients whose symptoms were deemed functional, 117 manifested the IBS symptoms of lower abdominal pain, cramping, and increased flatus. In contrast to adults, there appears to be an equal distribution of IBS in the pediatric population.

IBS is generally regarded as a chronic relapsing condition (Collins, 1999). In most patients, the presence and severity of IBS symptoms fluctuate over time. Though some reports suggest that 80% of patients are symptom-free at 5 years, other studies contradict this finding (Svendsen, Munck, & Anderson, 1985). One possible explanation is that IBS symptoms do not disappear altogether, but that patients may tend to respond to different sites and types of abdominal pain at different times (American Digestive Health Foundation, 2001). The dominance of abdominal pain, coexisting psychological difficulties, or multiple abdominal surgeries (e.g., choleccystectomy, appendectomy, hysterectomy) are factors associated with poor prognosis (Collins, 1999).

CLINICAL EVALUATION

A history of abdominal pain and disordered defecation that meet diagnostic criteria, along with a normal medical history and physical exam, support the diagnosis of IBS. A nutritional history can be useful to assess for caffeine, fructose, sorbitol, and other intake which might contribute to pain, bloating, or diarrhea. Some patients require diagnostic testing (e.g., sigmoidoscopy, colonoscopy, barium enema) to exclude other medical conditions, but such evaluation is not necessary for the majority of patients. In fact, superfluous testing may create additional anxiety and lead to unnecessary costs and risks. Limited laboratory screening may include complete blood count, erythrocyte sedimentation rate, stool studies, and breath hydrogen testing. If a patient has IBS, the results of these tests will essentially be negative. The presence of "red flag" warning signs (e.g., nocturnal pain, persitent vomiting, dysphagia, hematemesis, blood in stool) warrant more medical evaluation. In the absence of this evidence, the degree of functional impairment, parental concerns, and the physician's fear of a missed diagnosis influence the extent of evaluation (Hyams, 1999). The differential diagnosis of IBS requires consideration of the following categories of disease conditions: (1) dietary factors (e.g., lactose, caffeine, alcohol); (2) infection, bacterial or parasitic; (3) inflammatory bowel diseases, such as Crohn's disease or ulcerative colitis; (4) psychiatric dysfunction; (5) malabsorptive disorders; and (6) miscellaneous disease conditions, including endometriosis, Zollinger-Ellison syndrome and other endocrine tumors, and HIV-related diseases. It is important to note that IBS may coexist with some of these conditions, such as an inflammatory bowel disease.

Our psychosocial assessment includes a pain and IBS symptom history, review of diagnostic criteria, and evaluation of social-emotional contributors. Particular attention is given to factors that precipitate or maintain IBS symptoms and poor levels of daily functioning. The assessment is similar to the evaluation of RAP (see Chapter 6) and consistent with the biopsychosocial model of IBS. To that end, we utilize a number of checklists and questionnaires as a means of gathering relevant clinical data. These may include but are not limited to measures of stress (Adolescent Perceived Events Scale—Abbreviated Version: Compas, Davis, Forsythe, & Wagner, 1987), coping (Responses to Stress Questionnaire: Connor-Smith Compas, Wadsworth, Thomsen, & Saltzman, 2000), emotional/behavior problems (Child Behavior Checklist: Achenbach, 1991), functional disability (Functional Disability Inventory: Walker & Greene, 1991), and parental/familial beliefs about and responses to pain/GI symptoms (Illness Behavior Encouragement Scale—Revised: Walker & Zeman, 1992). A daily log of the frequency and severity of the child's primary IBS symptoms (e.g., abdominal pain, diarrhea, distention) provides initial assessment data as well as a means of evaluating treatment response.

TREATMENT

To date, no cure for IBS has been found. Current treatment approaches are aimed at providing effective reassurance and symptom relief. Drossman and Thompson (1992) recommended a graduated, multicomponent treatment approach in which the amount and types of treatment are based on the severity of the IBS. They estimated that 70% of patients with IBS have mild symptoms. These patients have intermittent symptoms, no significant functional disability, and no serious pychological problems. For these patients, education about the pathophysiology of IBS, reassurance of the nonserious nature of the disorder, and dietary changes are indicated. Food and drink associated with symptom worsening are eliminated. For many patients, the restrictions will include coffee/caffeine, alcohol, fatty foods, and dairy products. About 25% of patients are estimated to have moderate IBS, characterized by intermittent disruptions in daily activities (e.g., missing work or school) and psychological distress. The use of a symptom diary to log diet, stressors, and symptoms is recommended. Behavioral treatments, like relaxation therapy, hypnosis, biofeedback, and cognitive-behavioral therapy, are suggested to help patients better cope with their symptoms. In some cases, certain medications may be recommended for relief of symptoms like abdominal pain, diarrhea, or constipation. Because of the chronic nature of IBS, negative drug side effects, initial placebo response, and the fact that no particular medication is of proven benefit in IBS per se, medication use is cautioned. The remaining 5% of patients have severe IBS, characterized by chronic pain, significantly impaired functioning, and serious psychological difficulties, such as depression, anxiety, personality disorder, or a history of major loss or abuse. These patients are typically seen at tertiary care centers and utilize health care services heavily. Antidepressants, including tricyclics (e.g., amitriptyline, desipramine) or selective serotonin reuptake inhibitors (e.g., fluoxetine), are recommended for central analgesia. A strong physician-patient working relationship, which may include physician-based behavioral techniques, is deemed essential. Consistent with these recommendations, Whitehead et al. (2004) reported that the IBS treatments employed most frequently were dietary advice, explanation, exercise advice, reassurance, advice to reduce stress, and antispasmodic treatments. Education and lifestyle were emphasized more than drugs.

Jailwala, Imperiale, and Kroenke (2000) completed a systematic review of randomized, controlled trials of pharmacological agents for adult IBS. The 70 studies selected were randomized, double-blind, placebo-controlled, parallel, or crossover trials of a pharmacologic intervention for adult patients. The most common medication classes were smooth muscle relaxants, bulking agents, prokinetic agents, psychotropic agents, and loperamide. The strongest evidence for efficacy was shown by smooth muscle relaxants for patients with abdominal pain as the predominant symptom. Loperamide seems to reduce diarrhea, but does not relieve abdominal pain. Evidence for use of psychotropic agents has been promising but inconclusive.

In terms of psychological treatment, Blanchard and Scharff (2002) reviewed 21 randomized controlled trials for adults. These studies evaluated brief psychodynamic psychotherapy, hypnotherapy, and various combinations of cognitive and behavioral interventions. Hypnotherapy emerged with the strongest evidence base, including superiority to a placebo control (Whorwell, Prior, & Faragher, 1984), good follow-up (Whorwell, Prior, & Colgan, 1987), and replication of results at two other sites (Galovski & Blanchard, 1998; Harvey, Hinton, Gunary, & Barry, 1989). Cognitive therapy had the next strongest results, including superiority to a placebo control and supportive evidence from three separate studies. A limitation was the fact that all of the cognitive therapy studies had been conducted by Blanchard and his colleagues at their Albany, New York, site. Since the publication of their article, a randomized, controlled, multicenter trial of 431 adults with moderate to severe symptoms (Drossman et al., 2003) has provided additional support for cognitive therapy. Finally, two trials provided support for brief psychodynamic psychotherapy (Svedlund, Sjodin, Ottosson, & Dotevall, 1983; Guthrie, Creed, Dawson, & Tomenson, 1993). These studies were conducted at separate sites, and both yielded results that have held up at a 1-year follow-up. Various other cognitive and behavioral therapies have also been evaluated, with mixed support.

To our knowledge, there have been no randomized, controlled trials examining IBS treatments for children and adolescents. Despite the absence of empirical support, the various pharmacological therapies used with adults are often used in pediatric populations. The strong evidence base for psychological or behavioral treatments for recurrent abdominal pain (Sanders et al., 1989; Finney, Lemanek, Cataldo, Katz, & Fuqua 1989) and toileting difficulties in children (Cox, Sutphen, Borowitz, Kovatchev, & Ling, 1998; Stark et al., 1997) suggests promise for the use of these therapies for pediatric IBS. Clearly, an important research priority will be randomized, controlled evaluations of pharmacological, psychological, and other treatment strategies for pediatric populations.

SUGGESTED TREATMENT PROGRAM

In our practice, we utilize a multicomponent treatment approach that includes education and reassurance, dietary modification, pharmacotherapy for symptom relief, and central analgesia and behavioral treatment. Our dietary and pharmacological strategies are consistent with Drossman and Thompson (1992) and overlap with those described in Chapter 6 on recurrent abdominal pain. In terms of behavioral treatment, we have developed a more focused cognitive-behavioral treatment program that is modeled after Blanchard's empirically supported treatment program for adults (Blanchard & Schwarz, 1987; Neff & Blanchard, 1987) and consistent with a biopsychosocial conceptualization of IBS (Drossman, 1998). Specifically, the program targets misinformation about IBS, chronic overarousal, and inability to manage stress and anxiety effectively. Program components include: (1) information and education about IBS, (2) pain behavior management training for parents, (3) relaxation training, (4) skin temperature biofeedback, and (5) stress management training. For many patients, we utilize the entire eight-session protocol. Some patients, however, benefit from a more focused approach, emphasizing their particular areas of need over others. As warranted, specific toileting skills training is offered. For example, the patient with constipation-predominant IBS may be instructed to sit on the toilet for 10 minutes after every meal and practice external anal sphincter strengthening exercises to prevent overflow incontinence.

The following are brief descriptions of our behavioral treatment components as well as a session-by-session outline of the entire protocol:

1. Information and education about IBS are provided in the effort to clarify misconceptions and allay concerns. Questions such as "What is IBS?" "What causes it?" "How is it diagnosed?" "Is it stress related?" and "How is it treated?" are answered. Patients and families are reassured that their pain and symptoms are real, but that no serious medical causes or physical cure exists. A biopsychosocial conceptualization of IBS is presented, and the rationale for behavioral treatment components is provided.

2. Pain behavior management training is offered to promote effective strategies for interacting with children in pain and minimize inadvertent reinforcement for pain behaviors. Parents are coached to reinforce their children for practice and use of coping strategies, normal patterns of daily activity, and school attendance. The importance of discouraging pain-related problem and avoidance behaviors is emphasized. Pain behavior management guidelines are tailored to meet specific patient and family needs, and formal reward/reinforcement programs are implemented as necessary.

3. Relaxation training emphasizes several increasingly brief relaxation strategies. These include progressive muscle relaxation, passive muscle relaxation, and cue-controlled relaxation. Relaxation training teaches children to monitor their physiological state and effect a relaxation response when needed. Home practice is required, and behavioral procedures to promote compliance with practice are implemented as needed.

4. Skin temperature biofeedback assists children in acquiring relaxation skills and provides a more direct means of learning to attenuate sympathetic arousal. At a cognitive level, biofeedback is incorporated to enhance children's perceptions of physiological control. As with relaxation training, home practice is required, and behavioral procedures to promote compliance with practice are implemented as needed.

5. Stress management training emphasizes two particular sets of strategies: (1) modification of stress-provoking thoughts that can trigger pain and other IBS symptoms and (2) development of five-step and means-end problem-solving skills as ways of actively coping with life stressors. Specifically, patients are trained to identify stressful thoughts and substitute coping self-statements. They are also taught strategies for handling immediate problems better and planning/attaining long term goals.

SESSION 1. Information and Education about IBS/Review of Psychological Assessment Behavior Management Guidelines for Parents

SESSION 2: Progressive Muscle Relaxation

SESSION 3: Passive Muscle Relaxation/Skin Temperature Biofeedback

SESSION 4: Cue Controlled Relaxation/Skin Temperature Biofeedback

SESSION 5: Review of Behavior Management Guidelines for Parents/ Cognitive Therapy: Changing Negative, Stress-Related Thoughts

SESSION 6: Cognitive Therapy: Changing Negative, Stress-Related Thoughts

SESSION 7: General and Social Problem-Solving Training

SESSION 8: General and Social Problem-Solving Training

REFERENCES

Achenbach, T. M. (1991). *Manual for the Child Behavior Checklist 14-18 and 1991 Profile.* Burlington, VT: University of Vermont Department of Psychiatry.

American Digestive Health Foundation. (2001). *Irritable bowel syndrome: Part 1: Nosology, epidemiology, and pathophysiology.* Bethesda, MD: American Digestive Health Foundation.

Bennett, E. J., Tennant, C. C., Piesse, C., Badcock, C-A., & Kellow, J. E. (1998). Level of chronic life stress predicts clinical outcome in irritable bowel syndrome. *Gut, 43,* 256–261.

Blanchard, E. B., & Scharff, L. (2002). Psychosocial aspects of assessment and treatment of irritable bowel syndrome in adults and recurrent abdominal pain in children. *Journal of Consulting and Clinical Psychology, 70,* 725–738.

Blanchard, E. B., & Schwarz, S. P. (1987). Adaptation of a multicomponent treatment program for irritable bowel syndrome to a small group format. *Biofeedback, 12*, 63–69.

Collins, S. M. (1999). Natural history and prognosis. In R. Stockbrugger, & F. Pace (Eds.), *The irritable bowel syndrome manual* (pp. 81–86). London, UK: Mosby-Wolfe.

Compas, B. E., Davis, G. E., Forsythe, C. J., & Wagner, B. M. (1987). Assessment of major and daily life events during adolescence: The Adolescent Perceived Events Scale. *Journal of Consulting and Clinical Psychology, 55*, 534–541.

Connor-Smith, J. K., Compas, B. E., Wadsworth, M. E., Thomsen, A. H., & Saltzman, H. (2000). Responses to stress in adolescence: Measurement of coping and involuntary stress responses. *Journal of Consulting and Clinical Psychology, 68*, 976–992.

Cox, D. J., Sutphen, J., Borowitz, S., Kovatchev, B., & Ling, W. (1998). Contribution of behavior therapy and biofeedback to laxative therapy in the treatment of pediatric encopresis. *Annals of Behavioral Medicine, 20*, 70–76.

Drossman, D. A. (1998). Presidential address: Gastrointestinal illness and the biopsychosocial model. *Psychosomatic Medicine, 60*, 258–267.

Drossman, D. A. (1999). An integrated approach to the irritable bowel syndrome. *Aliment Pharmacology Therapy, 13*(Suppl. 2), 3–14.

Drossman, D. A., & Thompson, G. (1992). The irritable bowel syndrome: Review and a graduated multicomponent approach. *Annals of Internal Medicine, 116*, 1009–1016.

Drossman, D. A., Toner, B. B., Whitehead, W. E., Diamant, N. E., Dalton, C. B., Duncan, S., Emmott, S., Proffitt, V. Akman, D., Frusciante, K., Le, T., Meyer, K., Bradshaw, B., Mikula, K. Morris, C. B., Blackman, C. J., Hu, Y., Jia, H., Li, J. Z., Koch, G. G., Bangdiwala, S. I. (2003). Cognitive-behavioral therapy versus education and desipramine versus placebo for moderate to severe functional bowel disorders. *Gastroenterology, 25*, 249–253.

Drossman, D. A., Whitehead, W. E., & Camilleri, M. (1997). Irritable bowel syndrome: A technical review for practice guideline development. *Gastroenterology, 112*, 2120–2137.

Drossman, D. A., Zhiming, L., Andruzzi, E., Temple, R. D., Talley, N. J., Thompson, W. G., Whitehead, W. E., Janssens, J., Funch-Jensen, P., Corazziari, E., & Richter, J. E. (1993). U. S. Householder Survey of Functional Gastrointestinal Disorders: Prevalence, Sociodemography, and Health Impact. *Digestive Diseases and Sciences, 38*, 1569–1580.

Everhart, J. E., & Renault, P. F. (1991). Irritable bowel syndrome in office-based practice in the United States. *Gastroenterology, 100*, 998–1005.

Finney, J. W., Lemanek, K. L., Cataldo, M. F., Katz, H. P., & Fuqua, R. W. (1989). Pediatric psychology in primary health care: Brief targeted therapy for recurrent abdominal pain. *Behavior Therapy, 20*, 283–291.

Galovski, T. E., & Blanchard, E. B. (1998). The treatment of irritable bowel syndrome with hypnotherapy. *Applied Psychophysiology and Biofeedback, 23*, 219–232.

Gaynes, B. N., & Drossman, D. A. (1999). The role of psychosocial factors in irritable bowel syndrome. *Balliere's Clinical Gastronenterology, 13*, 437–452.

Guthrie, E., Creed, F., Dawson, D., Tomenson, B. (1993). A randomised controlled trial of psychotherapy in patients with refractory irritable bowel syndrome. *British Journal of Psychiatry, 163*, 315–321.

Hahn, B. A., Yan, S., & Strassels, S. (1999). Impact of irritable bowel syndrome on quality of life and resource use in the United States and United Kingdom. *Digestion, 60*, 77–81.

Harvey, R. F., Hinton, R. A., Gunary, R. M., & Barry, R. E. (1989). Individual and group hypnotherapy in treatment of refractory irritable bowel syndrome. *Lancet, I*, 424–425.

Hyams, J. S. (1999). Chronic and recurrent abdominal pain. In P. E. Hyman (Ed.), *Pediatric functional gastrointestinal disorders* (pp. 7.1–7.21). New York: Academic Professional Information Services.

Hyams, J. S., Burke, G., Davis, P. M., Rzepski, B., & Andrulonis, P. A. (1996). Abdominal pain and irritable bowel syndrome in adolescents: A community-based study. *Journal of Pediatrics, 129*, 220–226.

Hyams, J. S., Treem, W. R., Justinich, C. J., Davis, P., Shoup, M., & Burke, G. (1995). Characterization of symptoms in children with recurrent abdominal pain: Resemblance to irritable bowel syndrome. *Journal of Pediatric Gastroenterology and Nutrition, 20,* 209–214.

International Foundation for Functional Gastrointestinal Disorders (IFFGD). (2002). *IBS in the real world survey: Summary findings.* Milwaukee: Author.

Jailwala, J., Imperiale, T. F., & Kroenke, K. (2000). Pharmacological treatment of the irritable bowel syndrome: A systematic review of randomized, controlled trials. *Annals of Internal Medicine, 133,* 136–147.

Manning, A. P., Thompson, W. E., Heaton, K. W., & Morris, A. F. (1978). Towards a positive diagnosis of the irritable bowel. *British Medical Journal, 2,* 653–654.

Neff, D. F., & Blanchard, E. B. (1987). A multi-component treatment for irritable bowel syndrome. *Behaviour Therapy, 18,* 70–83.

Physician Drug and Diagnosis Audit (PDDA). (1999). Newton, PA: Scott-Levin PMSI Inc.

Rasquin-Weber, A., Hyman, P. E., Cucchiara, S., Fleisher, D., R., Hyams, J. S., Milla, P. J. et al. (1999). Childhood functional gastrointestinal disorders. *Gut, 45*(Suppl. II), II60–II68.

Sanders, M. R., Rebgetz, M., Morrison, M., Bor, W., Gordon, A., Dadds, M. et al. (1989). Cognitive-behavioral treatment of recurrent nonspecific abdominal pain in children: An analysis of generalization, maintenance, and side effects. *Journal of Consulting and Clinical Psychology, 57,* 294–300.

Sandler, R. S. (1990). Epidemiology of irritable bowel syndrome in the Unitedn States. *Gastroenterology, 99,* 409–415.

Stark, L.. J., Opirari, L. C., Donaldson, D. L., Danovsky, M. B., Rasile, D. A., & DelSanto, A. F. (1997). Evaluation of a standard protocol for retentive encopresis. *Journal of Pediatric Psychology, 22,* 619–633.

Svedlund, J., Sjodin, I., Ottosson, J. O., & Dotevall, G. (1983). Controlled study of psychotherapy in irritable bowel syndrome. *Lancet, 2,* 589–592.

Svendsen, J. H., Munck, L. K., & Andersen, J. R. (1985). Irritable bowel syndrome prognosis and diagnostic safety: A 5-year follow-up study. *Scandinavian Journal of Gastroenterology, 20,* 415–418.

Thompson, W. G., Longstreth, G. F., Drossman, D. A. , Heaton, K. W., Irvine, E. J., & Muller-Lissner, S. A. (1999). Functional bowel disorders and functional abdominal pain. *Gut, 45,* 1143–1147.

Thompson, W. G., Longstreth, G. F., Drossman, D. A., Heaton, K., Irvine, E. J., & Muller-Lissner, S. (2000). Functional bowel disorders and functional abdominal pain. In D. A. Drossman, E. Corraziari, N. J. Talley, & W. E. Whitehead (Eds)., *Rome II. The functional gastrointestinal disorders: Diagnosis, pathophysiology, and treatment – A multinational consensus* (2nd ed., pp. 351–432). McLean, VA: Degnon Associates.

Walker, L. S., & Greene, J. W. (1991). The Functional Disability Inventory: Measuring a neglected dimension of child health status. *Journal of Pediatric Psychology, 16,* 39–58.

Walker, L. S., Guite, J. W., Duke, M., Barnard, J. A., & Greene, J. W. (1998). Recurrent abdominal pain: A potential precursor of irritable bowel syndrome in adolescents and young adults. *Journal of Pediatrics, 132,* 1010–1015.

Walker, L. S., & Zeman, J. L. (1992). Parental response to child illness behavior. *Journal of Pediatric Psychology, 17,* 49–71.

Wells, N. E., Hahn, B. A., & Whorwell, P. J. (1997). Clinical economics review: Irritable bowel syndrome. *Alimentary Pharmacology and Therapeutics, 11,* 1019–1030.

Whitehead, W. E., Levy, R. L., Von Korff, M., Feld, A. D., Palsson, O. S., Turner, M., & Drossman, D. A. (2004). The usual medical care for irritable bowel syndrome. *Alimentary Pharmacology & Therapeutics, 20,* 1305–1315.

Whorwell, P. J., Prior, A., & Colgan, S. M. (1987). Hypnotherapy in severe irritable bowel syndrome: Further experience. *Gut, 28,* 423–425.

Whorwell, P. J., Prior, A., & Faragher, E. B. (1984). Controlled trial of hypnotherapy in the treatment of refractory irritable bowel syndrome. *Lancet,* 1232–1234.

Defecation Disorders | 8

Defecation disorders such as retentive fecal incontinence (RFI) and stool toileting refusal are common childhood problems that require significant health care resources. Estimates report that children with defecation disorders comprise 3% to 10% of all general pediatric visits and 25% to 30% of all pediatric gastroenterology visits (Fishman, Rappaport, Schonwald, & Nurko, 2003; Hatch, 1988; Youssef & DiLorenzo, 2001). These problems can cause pain, discomfort, and anguish for children. Families find these disorders shameful and difficult to manage, and, in addition, they are often a source of conflict between children and parents due to common misconceptions about the etiology of the problem. A unique feature of fecal incontinence is the isolation that children and families experience: they typically report knowing no one else with this problem. Families can avoid such distress, however, as fecal incontinence is a condition that is very amenable to treatment.

PATHOPHYSIOLOGY OF NORMAL DEFECATION: THE INTERACTIVE NATURE OF PHYSIOLOGY AND BEHAVIOR

Normal defecation requires the coordination of physical and behavioral functions. In order to understand the problems associated with defecation, it is also important to understand the specific functions of normal defecation. The pathway of the physiological functions begins with the gastrocolic reflex that occurs after eating. Eating triggers peristalsis or the movement of the food through the gastrointestinal (GI) tract. Typically, once food leaves the mouth and begins its descent into the gut, we lose consciousness of the process of digestion: the enteric nervous system (ENS) is in charge.

The colon is a muscular organ which absorbs more than 90% of the fluid that enters it. It is estimated that although digested food takes less than 2 hours to reach the colon, it may take as long as 2–5 days for it to be expelled as stool. A change from liquid to semisolid occurs in the right transverse portion of the colon. The descending colon serves as a conduit through which stool passes to the rectum, a storage area where further absorption occurs. Filling and distension of the rectum result in: (1) increased colonic peristalsis, (2) reflexive relaxation of internal anal sphincters, and (3) the sensation to defecate, which is recognized through the stretch receptors in the rectal tissue. The external anal sphincter then contracts to maintain continence

(McGrath, Mellon, & Murphy, 2000; Whitehead, Parker, Masek, Cataldo, & Freeman, 1981).

Mechanisms that control defecation are in place in the newborn. It is usually during the time of toilet training that the process of defecation is no longer reflexive and the control of the anal sphincter muscle is learned and becomes a conscious decision (Gershon, 1998).

Behaviors necessary for learning to use the toilet include the ability to pay attention to bodily cues: "listening to the body," understanding the appropriate versus inappropriate places for stooling, and having the motivation to act on these functions. Additionally, for typically developing children, the ability to undress and to get to the toilet is necessary. Once on the toilet, for typically to strain to initiate defecation. Finally, the child needs to be able to clean him- or herself up.

Problems with toileting occur when functions in either the physical or the behavioral domain are disrupted or when the coordination of the physiological and behavioral functions is not synchronized. Successful treatment of defecation problems requires an understanding of the physiology of digestion and elimination and an appreciation of the interaction between the brain and gut.

SPECIFIC DEFECATION DISORDERS

Infant Dyschezia

Infant dyschezia is defined by the multinational Rome Working Team (Rasquin-Weber et al., 1999) as "at least 10 minutes of straining and crying before successful passage of soft stools in an otherwise healthy infant less than 6 months of age" (p. 8). Infant dyschezia is a delay in the infant's learning to defecate; the infant has not coordinated the increase in intra-abdominal pressure with pelvic floor relaxation (Hyman, 1988). Clinical features include the baby turning red in the face and screaming in pain before defecation and stools that are free of blood. Episodes occur several times daily, for up to 20 minutes at a time. Infant dyschezia is outgrown during infancy and is resolved spontaneously when improved muscle coordination is achieved (Hyman, 1988).

No specific diagnostic tests are required. The key to differentiating between normal straining and infant dyschezia is the prolonged nature of the straining, fussing, or crying associated with straining. In addition, the child's stools are soft (Bishop, 2003). Treatment consists of reassurance to parents that this phenomenon is part of the infant's learning process, and anecdotal reports suggest that no intervention other than comforting the infant is needed (Youssef & DiLorenzo, 2001).

Fecal Incontinence

The broad definition of fecal incontinence is stooling in an inappropriate place. Weissenberg first defined the term encopresis in 1929. He described children with true psychogenic soiling, "the passage of whole bowel movements in the underwear or an abnormal place" (p. 55). Many gastroenterologists recognized that this explanation was insufficient at best. Levine (1975) broadened the definition to include a differentiation between those children who soiled because of constipation and stool retention, and children for whom the problem was not related to constipation.

However, a differentiation between fecal incontinence due to constipation and fecal incontinence consequently due to the absence of constipation was not made in the DSM-IV until 1994 (APA, 1994). Many pediatricians trained during this time period attributed fecal incontinence to psychological or behavioral problems, and patients were often referred to mental health professionals.

Although a distinction between children who have fecal incontinence due to medical problems or developmental delay and those whose incontinence is not due to organic causes other than idiopathic constipation has been established, the general term encopresis remains the predominant term in the literature. This nonspecific label has caused confusion with respect to both the etiology and the treatment of fecal incontinence.

Although fecal incontinence is easily identified, issues of subtyping of fecal incontinence are complicated. Lack of agreement regarding subtypes has contributed to discrepancies regarding prevalence, etiology, assessment, and treatment (McGrath et al., 2000). As with many attempts to impose theoretical constructs on behaviors, the subtyping of defecation disorders may vary from clinical experience.

McGrath et al. (2000) clarified the relationship between constipation and soiling. They reported that approximately 85% of children with soiling have concomitant constipation; and of children with constipation, 35% of girls and 55% of boys have soiling. In their schema, not all children who have constipation have fecal incontinence, but the large majority of children with fecal incontinence have constipation. They suggest that the pooling together of constipated children, incontinent children, and a child with constipation and incontinence has prevented effective analysis of symptoms and evaluation of differential outcomes. They view the term encopresis as one that does not aid in clear identification of symptomatology and they recommend using the labels fecal incontinence with constipation versus fecal incontinence to avoid confusion.

Other subtyping models have been proposed. Loening-Baucke (2002) corroborates the importance of distinguishing between those children with fecal incontinence resulting from an organic medical condition or the intake of medication versus those children for whom there is no organic

TABLE 8.1. Classifications of Fecal Incontinence

A. Fecal Incontinence Due to Medical Disorders

B. Retentive Fecal Incontinence (RFI)
   Primary
   Secondary

C. Nonretentive Fecal Incontinence (NRFI)
   Primary
   Secondary

---

etiology that has the broad "functional encopresis" label. Walker (2002) identifies three subtypes: manipulative soiling, soiling due to stress-induced diarrhea and loose bowels, and retentive encopresis based on chronic constipation.

Table 8.1 is a paradigm that presents a synthesis of information culled from the literature on defecation disorders and from 20 years of the first author's clinical experience. This model categorizes defecation disorders so that diagnosis/assessment is simplified with the goal of providing more effective treatment outcomes. This classification system recognizes medical issues at the same time allowing for the reciprocal impact of behavioral issues on these disorders.

SUBTYPES OF FECAL INCONTINENCE

Fecal Incontinence Due to Medical Disorders

The following outline delineates various medical conditions that can cause fecal incontinence (Felt, 1999). The medical problem may be due to neurological, structural malformations, endocrine disorders, or to drug side effects. Fecal incontinence also occurs as the result of a developmental delay or a developmental disorder.

1. **Neurological causes**
   a. Spinal cord abnormalities (tethered cord, myelomeningocele, spinal tumor)
   b. Hirschsprung's disease (congenital aganglionosis)

2. **Anorectal malformations**
   a. Imperforate anus
   b. Anterior ectopic anus
   c. Anteriorly located anus
   d. Anal stenosis
   e. Post-anal atresia repair

3. Endocrine disorders
   a. Hypothyroidism
   b. Diabetes insipidus
   c. Hypokalemia
   d. Uremia

4. Developmental/behavioral issues
   a. Autism spectrum disorder
   b. Developmental or cognitive delay

5. Drug side effects
   a. Anesthetiques or narcotics
   b. Anticholinergics
   c. Anticonvulsants

Retentive Fecal Incontinence (RFI)

The majority of children with fecal incontinence (ranging from 80% to 90%) present with retentive fecal incontinence (RFI) (Levine, 1975; Loening-Baucke, 1995; McGrath et al., 2000; Christophersen, 1991). The cycle typically begins with a painful bowel movement that leads to retention and the development of constipation. Although medical problems can cause constipation (see Figure 8.1), no obvious organic etiology is found in 90% to 95% of children with constipation. The most common cause of constipation in children is an interaction between psychological and physiological factors, a delay in defecation after experiencing a painful or frightening bowel movement. The child will hide, contract its buttocks and thighs, and stand in a stiff position with a preoccupied facial expression, or do what parents describe as "the potty dance." The urge to defecate is met with attempts to withhold: the child paradoxically contracts the muscles of the pelvic floor instead of relaxing them when straining to defecate. Stool retention and impaction stretch the colon over time and this is then associated with physiologic consequences, which include diminished sensory threshold at the rectum and weakened rectal sphincter musculature and colonic dysmotility (Felt et al., 1999.). The retention of feces becomes an acquired behavior, which is self-reinforcing because of the success in delaying defecation and in decreasing the child's anxiety that they will experience pain when stooling. Retentive fecal incontinence can easily become a chronic condition.

The DSM-IV (APA, 1994) uses the term encopresis for fecal incontinence. The criteria for a diagnosis of encopresis include:

1. The inappropriate passage of feces at least once a month for a minimum of the past 3 months.
2. A chronological or developmental age of at least 4 years.

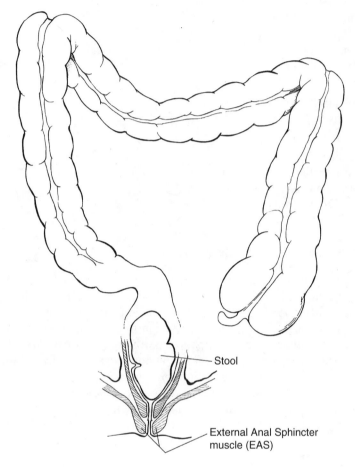

Stool

External Anal Sphincter
muscle (EAS)

FIGURE 8.1. Paradoxical contraction of external anal sphincter muscle: posterior view
(Drawing by Kathy Jung)

3. The problem cannot be due to a medical or physiological condition.
   Absence or presence of constipation and overflow incontinence
   should be noted.

The Rome international group (Rasquin-Weber et al., 1999) defined
functional fecal incontinence as occurring from infancy to 16 years of age
with a history of at least 12 weeks of:

1. Passage of large diameter stools at intervals less than 2 times per
   week.
2. Retentive posturing, that is avoiding defecation by purposively con-
   tracting the pelvic floor. As the pelvic floor muscles fatigue, the child
   uses the gluteal muscles, squeezing the buttocks together.

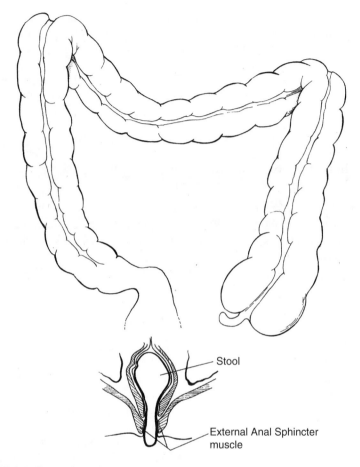

FIGURE 8.2. Relaxation of external anal sphincter muscle: posterior view (Drawing by Kathy Jung)

Nonretentive Fecal Incontinence (NRFI) or Stool Toileting Refusers

Nonretentive fecal incontinence (NRFI) occurs when children have not learned to stool on the toilet after achieving bladder control for a period of a month or longer. They stool on a regular basis without abdominal pain, constipation, or defecation, but they elect to defecate into a diaper, pull-up, or underwear (Brooks et al., 2000; Benninga, Bueller, Heymana, Tzgat, & Taminieu, 1994). Episodes of incontinence typically occur between 3 and 7 P.M. Children often report that "I was too busy playing outside to come in and use the toilet," or "I was in the middle of playing a game." The suggestion that these children deny or neglect their body's normal physical stimuli is often confirmed by a normal anorectal manometry function and normal colonic transit times using radio-opaque markers (Benninga & Taminiau, 2001).

NRFI in older children is more likely to be associated with psychiatric problems since these children appear unaware of the social consequences of their behavior on others. In the DSM-IV, NRFI is defined as encopresis in the absence of constipation.

The Rome international group (Rasquin-Weber et al., 1999) diagnostic criteria for functional nonretentive soiling is once a week or more for the preceding 12 weeks, in a child older than 4 years, a history of:

1. Defecation in places and at times inappropriate to the social context.
2. In the absence of structural or inflammatory disease.
3. In the absence of fecal retention.

Further subtyping of children with nonretentive fecal incontinence can include children with "toilet phobia," children who manipulate their environment using episodes on incontinence, and children who fail to reach this developmental milestone because of skill deficits such as not knowing how to stool sitting down (Kuhn, Marcus, & Pitner, 1999). These subcategories are not mutually exclusive.

Primary versus Secondary Fecal Incontinence

Another differentiation in subtyping of fecal incontinence in children is between primary versus secondary fecal incontinence, which can occur with both RFI and NRFI (Walker, 2002). Primary fecal incontinence refers to those children who have never been toilet trained: children who have reached 4 years of age without continence for a year. Secondary fecal incontinence refers to those children who have achieved independent bowel control for at least 1 year but then started having episodes of fecal incontinence. The first author's clinical experience has been that secondary FI (for both RFI and NRFI) can occur in response to either physical events (flu, bout of constipation) or in response to psychosocial stressors (birth of a sibling, divorce, or moving).

EPIDEMIOLOGY

Constipation Prevalence

The prevalence of constipation is important, since constipation is the cause of retentive fecal incontinence for a majority of children. Constipation is defined as the reduction in frequency of stools in this case because of the child's perception that the passage of stools which are hard will be difficult or painful (Levy & Volpert, 2004).

Recently, the Paris Consensus on Childhood Constipation Terminology (PACCT, 2005) Group found the Rome II criteria too restrictive. Consequently, they developed a working definition that would provide uniformity and facilitate discussions. The PACCT group defined constipation as the occurence of two or more of the following characteristics during the last 8 weeks:

    a. Frequency of bowel movements less than three per week
    b. More than one episode of fecal incontinence per week
    c. Large stools in the rectum or palpable on abdominal examination
    d. Passing of stools so large that they obstruct the toilet
    e. Retentive posturing and withholding behavior
    f. Painful defecation

Even if their stools are soft, children may withhold them and they may "feel" constipated. In children, minimal to mild constipation is frequent, transient, and recurrent, the peak incidence occurring between 2 to 4 years of age (Clayden, 1992). Research literature estimates that 3% of preschool-age children have problems with constipation, while 1% to 2% of school-age children have problems. The time from the onset of symptoms to diagnosis is 1 to 5 years (Loening-Baucke, 1993). Gender differences in constipation do not appear in the toddler years, but in school-age children, constipation is more prevalent in boys.

Fecal Incontinence

The statistics for fecal incontinence without specific subtyping are relatively consistent. Fishman et al. (2003) report a prevalence of 1% to 3% of the general pediatric population. Loening-Baucke (2002) cites the following prevalence: 8% for 4 year olds; 9% for 6 year olds; 6% for 10 to 11 year olds. Youssef and DiLorenzo (2001) state that 5% of children at the time of school entry have fecal incontinence, while McGrath et al. (2000) report a prevalence rate of 1.5% to 7.5% of school age children ages 6 to 12 years. Many researchers and clinicians believe fecal incontinence is underreported (Levine, 1975; Youssef & DiLorenzo, 2001; Loening-Baucke, 1989). The results of a recent population-based study in a multicultural population in the Netherlands indicate that only a small proportion of children with FI had seen a doctor for this problem: only 37.5% of 5–6 year olds and 27.4% of 11–12 year olds (Van Lehr, Bennigga, & Hirasing 2005). Table 8.2 presents data for epidemiology of subtypes of FI.

TABLE 8.2. Prevalence of Subtypes of Fecal Incontinence

Subtypes	Percentage of Children
1. FI due to medical/developmental disorders	5% to 10% (approximately)
2. RFI	80% to 95% (Levine, 1975; Youssef & Lorenzo, 2001)
3. NRFI	5% to 20% (Kuhn, Marcus, & Pitner, 1999)

Other Distinguishing Features

The consensus among researchers and clinicians is that fecal incontinence occurs more often in boys. Luxem and Christopherson (1994) give a prevalence rate of 3 to 6 times more frequently in boys than girls, while Levine (1975) reports a ratio of boys to girls as 6 to 1. Approximately 30% of children with fecal incontinence simultaneously have problems with enuresis (Levine, 1975). There is no evidence that fecal incontinence is related to social class, birth order, or family size or age of the parents (Levine, 1975). Data are limited regarding the impact of sociocultural factors on fecal incontinence. Differences in the rates of fecal incontinence among different ethnic groups are difficult to assess, since differences may reflect variations in diet, timing of toilet training, and different types of toileting training practices.

Although the child abuse literature has described a possible connection between fecal incontinence and child abuse, data supporting this theory from pediatric and gastroenterology research is rare (Walker, 2002). Though anal penetration can cause problems with elimination due to damage to the anal sphincter muscles, the association between child abuse and fecal incontinence is more the exception and assumptions should not be made without a thorough evaluation (Brayden & Altemeier, 1989).

COURSE AND PROGNOSIS

Fecal incontinence declines in incidence with increasing age and becomes infrequent in adolescence and rare in adulthood (Levine, 1975). In typically developing children, the persistence of fecal incontinence beyond age 16 is unusual (Rex, Fitzgerald, & Goulet, 1992); however, this issue remains difficult to assess because of the lack of clear criteria for remission and cure. Rockney, McQuade, Days, Linn, and Alario (1996) reported that at follow-up, 87% of patients treated had shown improvement, yet, at 1 year posttreatment, a significant number of children still had episodes of fecal incontinence. The chance of complete remission increases over time. Risk factors that can impede successful treatment include: poor adherence, significant coexisting psychological factors (Hatch, 1988); learning disabilities, difficult time toilet training, teen occurrence, lack of associated constipation (Levine, 1975), and previous unsuccessful treatment or nonretentive encopresis (Rockney et al., 1996). Children with difficulty with sphincter relaxation are typically predictive of a poor response to laxatives: children with FI with normal sphincter tone are likely to improve quickly. Poor gastric motility also predicts a poorer response. Data have also indicated that adherence to a treatment program improves fecal incontinence in all children, but that coexisting behavior problems are likely to be associated with poorer treatment outcome (Loening-Baucke, 2002).

Data are not available in regard to the percentage of individuals who experienced constipation in childhood and who have problems as adults.

However, adults presenting with megacolon often report enduring problems with constipation since childhood (Loening-Baucke, 2002).

ETIOLOGY

The etiology of fecal incontinence is directly related to the subtype of fecal incontinence.

Fecal Incontinence Due to Medical Problems

In children whose medical problems result in fecal incontinence, the medical condition is the core contributory factor. Defecation problems in neurologically impaired children have been well documented (DiLorenzo, 1997). The cause of these problems is varied and can include poor defecatory effort, abnormal muscle tone and coordination, poor dietary fiber intake, immobility with delayed colonic transit, use of drugs with anticholinergic properties, and the long-term use of laxatives: factors that can often coexist (DiLorenzo, 1997). Groves (1982) reported no specific criteria for differentiating fecal incontinence from generalized developmental delay in a review of the literature of the treatment of fecal incontinence in individuals with developmental disorders. Children with spina bifida may not have the muscle ability to control defecation depending upon the location of the lesion in their spinal cords. Children with imperforate anus may have problems with sensation that can affect their "learning" when they have to stool. Children with developmental disorders such as developmental delay or an autism spectrum disorder are more likely to have fecal incontinence due to problems with cognition, motivation, or a lack of awareness of social cues. Children with severe developmental delay, which includes motor impairment, are more prone to resistant constipation, in addition to their developmental lag in learning the necessary steps to use the toilet (Levine, 1975). Behavioral issues, such as oppositional behavior, in children with medical problems can arise secondarily as a response to the treatment program.

Retentive Fecal Incontinence

Theories regarding the etiology of retentive fecal incontinence have had a varied course reflecting the spectrum of ideological viewpoints of gastrointestinal disorders during the 20th century, but they were not typically substantiated by data. In the DSM-III, all types of fecal incontinence, with the exception of children with Hirchsprung's disease, were included under the diagnosis of "functional encopresis." In 1994, the DSM-IV distinguished between children with constipation and stool overflow and those children with intentional incontinence. The recognition that fecal incontinence is the result of the effects of long-standing functional constipation for the large majority of children has replaced earlier theories of psychopathology as the etiology (Levine, 1982; Fishman, 2003).

The major etiological factor of retentive fecal incontinence is stool retention due to the fear of painful defecation or subsequent to a painful bowel movement, which leads to constipation (Brooks et al., 2000; Loening-Baucke, 1993; McGrath et al., 2000). Loening-Baucke (1993) reports that 68% to 86% of children with constipation experience pain with defecation. Many gastroenterologists note that children with stool retention demonstrate an altered rectosphincteric reflux in which the stool in the rectum elicits paradoxical contraction of the external anal sphincter (EAS) muscles rather than the normal relaxation response during the attempt to defecate (Borowitz, 2001; McGrath et al., 2000). This paradoxical contraction becomes habitual: the association of the bowel movements and pain becomes a conditioned aversive response. Parents often observe the child posturing, tightening their legs, turning red, stiffening, and "dancing around." This is an attempt by the child to squeeze the pelvic muscles and the external sphincter in order to force the stool back up and to relieve the feeling of urgency to stool. The child is typically unaware of this pattern, which contributes to difficulties in changing the behavior. Many parents do not recognize that sitting on the toilet can be a cue for the child to withhold stool. They become frightened that a physical problem is preventing the child from stooling, because they think that the child is trying to push the stool out, not hold it in. The most common consequence of the stool retention is the overflow soiling that occurs around a hard stool that has developed because the rectum becomes dilated and filled with large amounts of fecal material.

Contributory factors to stool retention in younger children include the introduction of cow's milk or solid food (McClung, Boyne, Heitlinger, 1993). In older children contributory factors may coincide with practical issues such as: unavailability of a toilet, unpleasant facility, lack of privacy, dietary factors, and psychosocial factors such as: moving, the birth of a sibling, or stress in the family (Levine, 1981).

Nonretentive Fecal Incontinence

The etiology of nonretentive fecal incontinence is usually multifactorial (Kuhn, Marcus, and Pitner, 1999; Benninga et al., 1994). NRFI occurs more often in boys, possibly the result of not having as many practice sits on the toilet because they urinate standing up. Evidence does not support that children with stool-toileting refusal have more behavioral problems than a group of age and sex-matched children who were successfully toilet trained; however, a trend of a more difficult temperament has been identified (Blum, 1997). Van der Plas et al. (1999) demonstrated behavioral problems in 35% of children with NRFI using the Child Behavior Checklist (Achenbach, 1991). However, children with initial abnormal behavioral scores showed significant improvement of behavioral problems after successful treatment of their NRFI. Loening-Baucke (2002) found no significant differences in total behavior scores between children with fecal soiling who had constipation/retention and those that did not.

DIAGNOSIS

A comprehensive assessment of the child from both medical and behavioral perspectives is necessary to diagnose fecal incontinence. The purpose of the assessment is to obtain information regarding the child's specific type of defecation disorder and to identify which specific medical or behavioral factors are preventing the child from reaching this developmental milestone. Table 8.3 gives an outline of assessments needed for determining the subtype of fecal incontinence.

Medical Assessment

Medical assessment of fecal incontinence begins with a history of the child's general health, dietary habits, and current medications. A review of the child's stooling patterns from infancy, current stooling frequency, stool size, and stool consistency are important diagnostic pieces of information. The child should be asked two important diagnostic questions: (1) Can you feel the bowel movement coming? (2) Can you stop and start the bowel movement when you want to?

Symptoms that accompany constipation should be explored, including the following physical complaints: abdominal discomfort, infrequent bowel movements, palpable abdominal mass, bowel-movement withholding, pain prior to defecation, poor appetite, weight loss, irritability, and lethargy.

Youssef and DiLorenzo (2001) recommend radiological studies to assess the degree of fecal retention and the need for disimpaction, and if the problem is severe or chronic, evaluation of segmental colonic transit time using

TABLE 8.3. Guidelines for Assessment of Pediatric Patients with Fecal Incontinence

Medical Assessment
1. Obtain medical history—including current medications and dietary history
2. Evaluate stooling habits (current and past)
3. Rule-out constipation

Psychosocial Assessment
1. Obtain developmental history—including review of toileting readiness criteria and socio-cultural values that may impact timing
2. Obtain description of child's stooling problem
3. Clarify parental/family socio-cultural expectations regarding toileting
4. Evaluate child's level of compliance
5. Review prior treatment attempts

swallowed radio-opaque markers. When concerns regarding Hirschsprung's disease (HD) exist, a rectal biopsy confirming the absence of intramural ganglion cells is the gold standard to rule out (HD).

The trends in assessment of fecal incontinence over the past 20 years include: a decrease in barium enemas from 14% to 5%, a steady rate at 2% to 3% of rectal biopsy to rule out Hirschsprung's disease, and a rise in the use of anorectal manometry in the past 5 years (Fishman et al., 2003).

Psychosocial Assessment

Awareness of the significant contribution of physical issues to fecal incontinence has affected how fecal incontinence is evaluated from a behavioral and psychological perspective. Fishman et al. (2003) reported that psychiatric evaluations for children with fecal incontinence before referral to a gastroenterology clinic have decreased from 25% to 14%. This change in referral patterns indicates that pediatricians may have increased awareness of the primarily physical rather than psychological causes of fecal incontinence.

The first step is to evaluate the child's current stooling patterns. The following questions can be used to elicit the information:

1. Is the child stooling daily or is the child withholding stool?
2. Has the child shown behavioral indications of stool retention, such as the stiffening of legs or dancing around?
3. Does the child have the prerequisite skills necessary—can the child get to the toilet, pull down pants, sit, and stool?
4. Can the child communicate that he or she needs to use the toilet?
5. What is the child's level of compliance or oppositional behavior? The behaviors contributing to this problem that need to be evaluated
6. What behavioral skills does the child have?
7. What toileting habits has the child established? What is the history of the child's toilet training? What methods have been used and what have been the child's responses?

Finally, information from caregivers regarding prior treatment needs to be obtained and reviewed.

Cox et al. (2003) have developed a scale for evaluating children with encopresis, the term they use for fecal incontinence. Their instrument, the Virginia Encopresis-Constipation Apperception Test (VECAT) has proven to be a reliable, valid, discriminating, and sensitive test. Bowel-specific problems appear to best differentiate children with and without encopresis.

Treatment

Although defecation disorders are common childhood problems, definitive criteria for determining when to seek treatment have not been established. General recommendations include: when constipation has lasted for more than 6 months despite treatment with a stool softener, when there is frequent soiling and distress, when there is doubt over the cause of the symptoms, and when there are concerns that the child's school and peer relationships are being affected.

Evidence-Based Treatment Modalities

There are few controlled studies evaluating the treatment methodologies of fecal incontinence; instead, most evidence comes from case control studies, well-designed cohort studies, and case reports from clinicians. Reviews of the treatment literature (Borowitz, 2001; Brooks et al., 2000; McGrath et al., 2000; Whitehead, 1992; Stark et al., 1997) have evaluated effective interventions in the treatment of fecal incontinence.

McGrath et al. (2000) analyzed the treatment literature for fecal incontinence. The authors reviewed 65 intervention articles for the treatment of constipation and encopresis. Twenty-three studies were excluded because they were single-case designs. Studies that included equivalent subcategories of interventions were grouped and compared and 42 studies were evaluated. The intervention protocol for each study was identified and coded according to Chambless criteria (Chambless et al., 1996). Results indicated that no well-established interventions have emerged to date.

1. *The medical intervention category*: including a combination of cleaning out with laxative maintenance, dietary recommendations, and sitting schedule did not meet the criteria for efficacy.
2. *Three biofeedback interventions meet efficacy category*: one for constipation and abnormal defecation dynamics (full medical intervention plus biofeedback for paradoxical contraction), two fit promising intervention criteria for constipation and abnormal defecation dynamics (full medical intervention plus biofeedback for paradoxical contraction), and two fit the promising intervention criteria for constipation and abnormal defecation dynamics (full medical intervention plus biofeedback for EAS strengthening, correction of paradoxical contraction, and home medical intervention without fiber recommendation, and positive reinforcement).
3. *Two extensive behavioral interventions plus medical intervention*: met efficacy criteria for constipation plus incontinence (medical intervention without laxative maintenance plus positive reinforcement, dietary education, goal setting, and skills building presented in small-group format fit criteria for a promising intervention; and positive reinforcement and skills building focused on relaxation of the EAS during defecation but without biofeedback, plus medical intervention met the probably efficacious criteria).

The authors recommended the need for greater clarity in sample descriptions and treatment protocols and that recovery be defined as no fecal episodes or a full remission from constipation.

Brooks et al. (2000) reviewed nine randomized and controlled studies involving school-age children and three noncontrolled studies with preschool children for treatment of encopresis, functional constipation, and stool-toileting refusal. Their analysis stressed the need to adopt standardized definitions of subtypes, remission, and treatment standards. Although the results are affected by the lack of standardized treatment among studies, they reported the following results:

1. Positive outcomes for children with encopresis being treated with medical/behavioral approaches.
2. No differences in results between biofeedback intervention and the medical/behavioral intervention 3 to 12 months after treatment in 5 out of 6 studies.
3. Preschool children with stool-toileting refusal who do not exhibit severe stool-withholding behaviors or constipation are treated with resolution within 6 months.
4. When preschool children with stool-toileting refusal exhibit problems with stool retention and constipation, a more intensive medical-behavioral approach is needed.

Borowitz (2001) compared the short- and long-term effects of three additive treatment protocols in children with retentive fecal incontinence. The results indicated that enhanced toilet training (intensive medical therapy plus behavioral therapy) resulted in statistically significant decreases in the daily frequency of soiling for the greatest number of children as compared to intensive medical therapy or anal sphincter biofeedback therapy alone.

Benninga & Taminiau (2001) reported that the treatment of children with NRFI with no other symptoms of constipation and a normal colonic transit time is difficult. The suggested therapy for children with NRFI includes parental and child education and support, a nonjudgmental approach to the problem avoiding accusatory statements, and the use of a reward-based toileting program. Benninga & Taminiau also reported that "biofeedback seems to play no or only a minor role in the treatment of these children (p. S43).

Alternative therapies for the management of fecal incontinence have included acupuncture and dietary interventions. The use of acupuncture as a treatment modality was documented in a study in which 5 weekly placebo acupuncture sessions were followed by 10 true acupuncture sessions performed in children with constipation with and without fecal incontinence. Bowel movement frequency increased in boys with true acupuncture. Bowel movement frequency increased in girls after the placebo acupuncture and increased further with true acupuncture. No outcome data are reported on the effect on fecal incontinence (Broide et al., 2001).

Parents place great importance on diet in the management of fecal incontinence. Although a clinical review of randomized controlled trials found no evidence that diet alone as a treatment modality is effective for the treatment of RFI (Robin, 2000), an increase in dietary fiber and water is part of most treatment recommendations. For children older than 2 years of age, it is recommended that they consume fiber in the daily amount of their age plus 5 grams (Hyams, 2002). A recent study indicated that only 50% of children without constipation consume recommended daily amounts of fiber and children with constipation consumed no more than 25% of the recommended amount (McClung et al., 1993).

In summary, evidence-based research indicates no documented, standardized comprehensive treatments for retentive fecal incontinence. However, there are data and general agreement as to what components are effective in the management of this common childhood problem (Borowitz, 2002). Research studies consistently identified the following issues:

1. The need for clear definitions of fecal incontinence subtypes, treatment protocols, and criteria for remission or recovery.
2. Medical/behavioral approaches are effective for children with retentive fecal incontinence. Research indicates that long-standing conventional treatment regimens, including education of the child and family, medical intervention, and behavioral therapy, have not been surpassed as a primary treatment modality (Mikkelson, 2001).
3. Biofeedback has been shown to decrease paradoxical contraction of the external anal sphincter muscles, but has not shown to add a significant positive effect in overall treatment. Although biofeedback may have a role for those children who exhibit abnormal defecatory dynamics, no significant benefit of biofeedback was observed in the large majority of randomized studies (Hatch, 1988; McGrath et al., 2000; Whitehead, 1992).
4. Behavioral modification has proven to be a critical factor in treating fecal incontinence (McGrath et al., 2000). Examples of typical behavioral interventions include: documentation of stool passage, practice sits, use of a stool for feet, and rewards for compliance with taking medicine and sitting times (Levine, 1975; Loening-Baucke, 2002; Youssef, 2001).
5. The need for controlled studies indicating which behavioral methods or parenting techniques are most effective for the treatment of nonretentive fecal soiling.

A PROPOSED TREATMENT PLAN FOR FECAL INCONTINENCE

1. Clinical Interviews

Clinical interviews serve a variety of functions including: (1) obtaining information in order to determine type of defecation disorder, (2) identifying environmental contingencies and circumstances that may have

contributed to the origin of the problem or its maintenance, and (3) providing data regarding the emotional-behavioral competencies of the child
and parents.

a. Meet with the Family or Caregiver

Form a treatment "team" with parents. Reassure parents about this problem and explain why it is critical to overcome any unnecessary shame or
embarrassment that they may be feeling. It is important to dispel myths
that stooling problems are the result of poor parenting or indicative of
psychopathology. These steps should be followed when conferencing with
parents:

1. Review with parents why they think their child has this problem.
2. Ask what interventions they have tried and what has been successful.
3. Provide opportunity to view videotapes of former patients and their
   families in order to decrease the isolation that families and children
   experience.

Dealing with this discussion in a matter-of-fact tone so that families are at
ease is critical and sets a tone for dealing with fecal incontinence in a direct
nonjudgmental manner.

Meet with the caregiver prior to the scheduled meeting with the child
to obtain a comprehensive history and to obtain general developmental
information and information about the child's specific toileting problem.
There are two aspects of fecal incontinence that need to be evaluated. The
first is *how* the child stools. The following questions can be used to obtain
the information:

1. Is your child stooling on a daily basis?
2. Does your child have large caliber stools?
3. Does your child strain when stooling?
4. Does your child have a history of constipation?
5. Does your child have a history of food allergies?
6. Does your child have many small, hard stools on a daily basis?
7. Is there a family history of constipation? Of other GI problems?

The second issue is *where* the child stools. To obtain this information, the
following questions are helpful:

1. Does your child stool in the toilet? If no, have they ever stooled in the
   toilet?
2. Does your child hide in another room when stooling?
3. Does your child use a pull-up or does he or she stool in his or her pants?
4. If your child has fecal incontinent episodes, where and when do they
   occur?

b. Meet with the Child

In your meeting with the child, it is critical to provide reassurance to the child, since many children are initially very anxious during the first visit. Describing your office as a "school" to learn how to use the toilet is helpful for many children. The fact that no medicine will be administered and no physical exams will be conducted is reinforced. Children find comfort in viewing pictures of those who "successfully graduated" and thank-you notes made by other children who have had the same problem.

The following questions, adjusted to the age and the level of cognitive functioning of the child, are very helpful:

1. Do you poop everyday or only once in a while?
2. Do you poop in a pull-up, your pants, or in the toilet?
3. Are you afraid that it will hurt when you poop?
4. Do you remember having a poop that hurt coming out?
5. Do you want to learn how to poop on the potty?
6. Do you poop standing up or sitting down?
7. Do you have stomach aches?

2. Educate the Child and the Family

It is then important to educate the family. Education of families about toileting problems, including specific types, the etiology, and treatment issues, is a critical factor in the treatment process. The first author gives parents a copy of the Jane Brody (1992) article that appeared in the *New York Times* that discusses toileting problems from a parental/caregiver perspective. I emphasize that the etiology of elimination disorders is rarely psychopathological, yet parental reactions *to* toileting problems can often contribute to the development of emotional and behavioral problems in children. I focus on the following behavioral and psychological issues with the patient and his or her family:

1. The subtype of fecal incontinence needs to be identified immediately so that treatment is effective.
2. Fecal incontinence is a chronic problem that patients and families deal with in isolation.
3. Despite the chronicity of this problem, fecal incontinence is highly treatable *if* the parents and child follow the treatment plan.
4. Medical management needs to be aggressive with retentive fecal incontinence.
5. Statistics indicate by 16 years of age fecal incontinence disappears.
6. Determine who else in the child's world needs to be educated regarding this problem.

7. Reinforce that psychological problems are rarely the cause of fecal incontinence; however, psychological problems can often *result* from having incontinence.

It is important to answer questions and stress that treatment works if children and parents are consistent with the prescribed plans. Introduce the concepts of a stooling diary and stress the importance of their keeping accurate records, since the information will be a cornerstone for the treatment of their child.

3. Assess the Type of Toileting Problem

The flow chart in Figure 8.4 is useful in determining the subtype of toileting problem. Correct assessment of the toileting problem is a critical step in the treatment process. Table 8.4 summarizes the treatments for fecal incontinence.

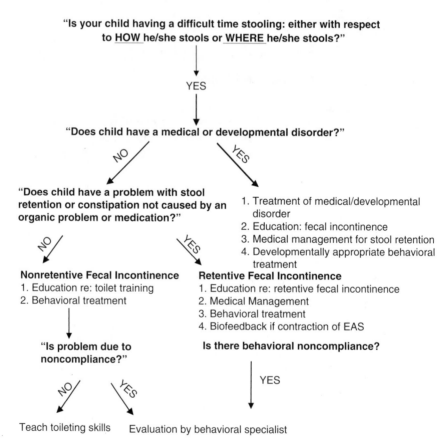

FIGURE 8.4. A summary of the treatment for fecal incontinence

TABLE 8.4. Treatment of Fecal Incontinence (FI) by Subtype

1. **Fecal Incontinence Due to Medical/Developmental Disorders**
   A. Identify the medical/behavioral problem affecting stooling
   B. Address developmental issues and behaviors affecting stooling
   C. Assess child's motivation, and issues that may impact compliance (e.g., oppositional behavior)
   D. Schedule regular follow-up visits

2. **Retentive Fecal Incontinence**
   A. Medical management by physician
      1. Determine if child is impacted/needs to be cleaned out
      2. Use stool softeners or laxatives if child is constipated
      3. If problems with compliance refer to behavioral specialist for evaluation
   B. Behavior management
      1. Explanations of digestion and elimination to child
      2. Implement structured behavioral toileting program
      3. Suggest increase in dietary fiber and water
      4. Treat non compliance and oppositional behavior if exists
      5. Schedule regular follow-up visits

3. **Nonretentive Fecal Incontinence**
   A. Implement structured behavioral toileting program
   B. Treat noncompliance and oppositional behavior if it exists
   C. Schedule regular follow-up visits

4. Treatment of Subtype of Fecal Incontinence

See Table 8.4 for specific components of treatment plan for subtypes.

PROPOSED TREATMENT FOR FECAL INCONTINENCE DUE TO MEDICAL/BEHAVIORAL PROBLEMS

Identify Medical/Developmental Issues

Clarify with the family the diagnosis of the medical or developmental problem. Medical issues need to be treated by the child's physician. Medical management of the fecal incontinence will vary according to the specific presenting physical problem. Information regarding what the child is physically capable of doing, for example: Can they walk to the toilet and are they cognitively capable of understanding? Does their medical or behavioral problem affect their being able to feel when they are going to have a bowel movement? It is important to collaborate with the with the child's physician so that medical and behavioral suggestions are consistent. For children with medical issues or special developmental needs, the toileting program should be a component of the child's 504 plan at school.

Address How Medical and Behavioral Problems Affect Stooling

Many medical and developmental problems can lead to fecal incontinence. Children with specific medical and developmental conditions that cause fecal incontinence need physician guidance regarding a medical plan that will maximize the child's ability to then follow a behavioral treatment plan. Without the coordination between medical and behavioral treatment plans the child will have difficulty achieving mastery over this critical developmental milestone. As with any behavioral plan, establishing good rapport and obtaining the patient's cooperation is a cornerstone of treatment.

For example, Hirschsprung's disease, an uncommon congenital abnormality of the pelvic sympathetic nervous system involving absence of ganglion cells from the distal rectum and a variable length of more proximal bowel (Hatch, 1988), is a cause of fecal incontinence in children. HD, occurring in 1 out of 5,000 live births, is more common in males. When symptoms are present since birth and there is delayed passage of meconium, the probability of HD is greater. Surgery is the definitive treatment for Hirschsprung's disease. The aganglionic bowel is resectioned. The distal 1 cm of sensitive anorectum is retained to allow for future continence and control of defecation (Hatch, 1988). A structured behavioral plan that includes (1) medical management, (2) practice sits, (3) teaching to strain, and (4) rewards for positive attempts is a necessary adjunct to medical treatment.

A child with spina bifida may not be able to feel when they need to stool depending on where the lesion in their spine is; however, a structured toileting program can help the child stay dry and clean thus increasing their self-esteem.

For children with autism spectrum disorders, a structured program is very effective. Making a social storybook of pictures taken in the child's home of the toilet, the bathroom, and the child sitting on the toilet is very helpful. Once the child "gets" the process there is often a very positive response. While in the office, children with autism spectrum disorder may appear not be listening and not interested, however, the combination of a structured sitting program using rewards and the toileting storybook has been very useful.

Treat Oppositional Behavior or Noncompliance with Treatment Plan

Some children may use the struggle over toileting issues to assert their need for independence or for control. If behavioral problems such as non-compliance or oppositional behavior exist and interfere with the child's following the behavioral plan, referral to a behavioral health specialist is recommended (Stark, Spirito, Lewis & Hart, 1990).

PROPOSED TREATMENT OF RETENTIVE FECAL INCONTINENCE

Medical Management

It is important to first determine if a child is impacted and needs to be cleaned out. A critical factor in dealing with a child with retentive fecal incontinence is ensuring a sufficient clean out. Some pediatricians are not aggressive with the initial bowel clean-out process. If this first step is not successfully accomplished, the child will not be able to be successful regardless of how compliant he or she is.

Disimpaction can either be by the oral route or the rectal route. Youssef and DiLorenzo (2001) suggest weighing the options with families and patients. Although the rectal route is typically more effective, some children and families are initially adverse to this method. In cases of severe impaction, an admission to the hospital for a GoLytely cleanout maybe warranted. If there is doubt about the effectiveness of a clean out, an X-ray is recommended (Youssef & DiLorenzo, 2001).

It is important to then proceed with a discussion of the child's previous medical care in dealing with this problem. Many pediatricians are very knowledgeable about toileting problems and others are more laissez-faire, telling parents that the child will outgrow the problem when he or she is ready.

Use of Stool Softeners or Laxatives

After a clean out has been accomplished, the next step is the prevention of the reaccumulation of stool by use of laxatives and stool softeners. A maintenance dose of laxatives or stool softeners needs to be prescribed by the physician so that during the process of behavioral intervention, stooling is not difficult for the child. Parents have concerns regarding the abuse of or the child's dependence on laxatives; however, when the parent and physician are monitoring the administration, this is unlikely to happen.

Laxatives can be classified in four broad categories: (1) bulking agents, (2) lubricating agents, (3) osmotic laxatives, and (4) stimulant laxatives (Levy & Volpert, 2004). Fiber, a nonabsorbable complex carbohydrate, is the best example of a bulking agent. Bulking agents hold on to water and soften the stool, making it easier to pass. Metamucil and Konsyl contain processed husk from psyllium, while Citrucel is based on methyl cellulose, a synthetic fiber. Fibercon, which is available in caplet form, is a complex, nonabsorbable starch-calcium polycarbophil.

Lubricating agents or stool softener which prevent the stool from becoming compacted and dry include mineral oil, Colace (docusate sodium), and Kondremul, a combination of fiber and mineral oil in emulsion form.

Osmotic laxatives increase the accumulation of water in the intestinal tract, preventing stools from drying, which facilitates more rapid transit. The most common osmotic laxatives include nonabsorbable magnesium salts (Milk of Magnesia, magnesium citrate), sodium phosphate (fleet phosphosoda), and Miralax, which contains polyethylene glucol 3350 (PEG). Anecdotal experience and recent research indicates that Miralax is a palatable and effective laxative because it has virtually no taste and it can easily be mixed in juice or water. None of the bulking or lubricating agents or the osmotic laxatives carry long-term side effects (Arora & Srinivasan, 2005). Research does not support parental concerns that mineral oil interferes with the absorption of vitamins in food.

Stimulant laxatives work by directly signaling the muscles and nerves of the intestine to contract and expel its content. These include Senokot (a derivative of the senna leaf) or alkaloid chemicals such as bisacidyl, Correctol, or Ducolax. Increasing may be necessary to produce the same stimulating effect, and therefore may be habit forming (Levy & Volpert, 2004).

Loening-Baucke (2002) conducted a prospective, randomized, controlled clinical study to determine the effectiveness of polyethylene glycol (PEG) 3350 for the treatment of constipation and fecal incontinence as compared to the use of Milk of Magnesia. Results indicated both therapies were effective in increasing the frequency of bowel movements and decreasing the number of incontinent occurrences. Miralax, the brand name for PEG 3350, proved to be a palatable, well-tolerated medication. Miralax was also compared to lactulose and the results of this study indicated that treatment of childhood constipation with PEG 3350 resulted in a significantly higher success rate, compared with lactulose therapy (Pashankar, Loening-Baucke, & Bishop, 2003). The first author's experience is that the use of Miralax has had a significant positive effect on medication compliance postcleanout.

Behavior Management

A behavioral plan for treatment of RFI with specific parts should be implemented. Begin with addressing the educational/cognitive component. An effective way to begin is by using pictures of the GI tract (see appendix C) and giving the child a simple explanation of digestion and elimination. I ask the child to tell me something that they like to eat and then pictorially show them what happens to that food in terms of digestion (food turning into poop). During the explanation, I will make a point of engaging the child in the discussion (e.g., What do we chew with?). The more involved the child is the more effective the message is. I will then show another GI and color the colon completely brown saying, "Some kids hold their poop inside and it gets stuck, does this ever happen to you?" I will then use another chart to show the child how the nerve endings in the rectum alert us to the fact that "the poop is ready to come out." I will show the nerve endings sending a message to the brain.

A behavioral modification plan is then created to promote positive steps toward specific goals agreed upon at each session. Focus is on the child as an active participant in his or her self-care. The behavioral plan needs to focus on a precise analysis of the child's current situation. It is important to differentiate between the goal of eliminating stool withholding (having the child evacuate on a regular basis) versus eliminating stooling in inappropriate places. For children with retentive fecal incontinence, the goal is have the child begin to stool on a regular basis—setting a goal of clean pants may only increase the stool retention. ***You need to start where the child is to maximize success***: ask the child what they think they can do to get to the goal. The following suggestions are presented to the child and parents:

1. Create a large poster with the use of stickers for successful completion of goals (e.g., taking medicine, having regular toilet sits). The goal is to enlist the child's cooperation in completing a specific toileting task. It is important to make the first task something the child can accomplish easily to foster a feeling of efficacy. The focus is on incremental improvement. Praise is an important component of success, but only for the completed task.

2. Parents need to be consistent with their charting of the stooling diary (see appendix A) and the medication. They should remind about sitting times, but not nag. Resistance will be dealt with in the doctor's office.

3. It is important to teach and practice how "to strain" in the doctor's office. We practice feeling the stomach muscles tighten as the child takes in a deep breath while keeping everything below his or her beltline relaxed. Parents are to place their hands on their child's legs to feel any tension. If tension is detected, then parents are to prompt the child to relax.

4. Routine practice toilet sits, usually 15 to 20 minutes after meals, are strongly suggested.

5. Cleanliness training of the child's own body and learning to clean his or her own pants is very important: the child needs to experience the consequences of his or her actions (Vitito, 1999).

6. Regular follow-up visits (20 to 30 minutes per visit) are scheduled. The first three or four visits are weekly to ensure that treatment plans are in place.

7. Children's toileting books are often a helpful adjunct to behavioral therapy (see appendix B).

Dietary Changes

Dietary changes, including an increase of fiber and water, are recommended. However, it is important to tell parents that data indicate that dietary changes alone have not been proven to be sufficient to treat RFI.

Treating Noncompliance

If noncompliance exists, it is important to talk with the child to see if one can determine the cause of the noncompliance, and consequences need to be enforced. Once the child is stooling regularly, the issues of control can be prominent. Have the parent make sure the routine is understood; that consequences are in place, and that the child is responsible for problems that arise.

Many times the issue becomes the parent's "problem," and the child appears immune to both the physical and psychological consequences of this behavior.

PROPOSED TREATMENT FOR NONRETENTIVE FECAL INCONTINENCE

Implement a Structured Behavioral Plan

The behavioral treatment plan for NRFI should consist of modeling and teaching reinforcement. Toilet refusing behavior should be addressed with a gradual shaping procedure. If the child is reluctant to sit on the toilet for practice sits, the parent may first begin with having the child wear a diaper and stool near the bathroom, then in the bathroom standing up, then squatting, and then sitting on the toilet with a diaper on. Kuhn, Marcus, and Pitner (1999) recommend that boys sit down and urinate to give them extra practice sits on the toilet. The goal is to establish a positive experience associated with sitting on the toilet.

Once the child is comfortable sitting on the toilet and there are no concerns regarding hard stools, regular sitting or scheduled prompting can occur. To take advantage of the gastrocolic reflex, sits should be scheduled 5 to 20 minutes after eating. Incentives or rewards can be helpful to reinforce age-appropriate toileting behaviors. However for most children, the sense of accomplishment that they feel in accomplishing their weekly goals is the biggest reward they can receive. Praising the child for "being a big kid" is also helpful. Consequences such as cleaning his or her own pants need to be established for episodes of incontinence.

Treat Noncompliance or Oppositional Behavior if It Exists

If fecal incontinence is due to resistance or noncompliance and not a result of a skill deficit, then referral to a pediatric psychologist or another mental health practioner is warranted. The following steps are recommended with children for whom noncompliance is due to oppositional behavior: identify potential unrealistic parental expectations, address the toilet refusal behavior with the child, ensure that the child's stools are soft and well formed, schedule prompted toilet sits, provide incentives for stooling and self-initiation, and arrange physician contact in case of stool withholding (Kuhn, Marcus, & Pitner, 1999; Taubman, 1997).

NEW DIRECTIONS

Ritterband et al. (2003) have reported a new medium for treating fecal incontinence. The study evaluated the benefits of enhanced toilet training delivered through the Internet for children with fecal incontinence. The children who participated in the web intervention demonstrated greater improvements in terms of reduced fecal soiling, increased defecation in the toilet, and increased unprompted trips to the toilet as compared to a group that received medical care but no intervention from the Internet. This new methodology may be appealing to some children.

PREVENTION

Prevention of defecation disorders begins with the education of pediatricians, pediatric psychologists, nurse practitioners, and behavioral pediatricians—health professionals who are providing primary care. Education should include concise recommendations regarding optimal feeding practices, toilet-training readiness markers, subtypes of toileting problems, and high-risk factors at different developmental time frames. Levine (1975) assessed factors that occur in infancy, toddlerhood, and at school age that can contribute to the development of a defecation disorder. The existence of one or more of these factors can alert the health care professional that the child may be at risk for the development of a defecations disorder. Education of school nurses and preschool teachers who will likely encounter young children with these problems is also recommended and so that they do not assume a psychological etiology for the problem.

Prevention is particularly relevant with respect to the avoidance of retentive fecal incontinence, since hard painful stools may occur as early as 1 year of age and early detection is critical. Recognizing the symptoms of constipation and intervening early can avoid physical and behavioral problems from developing. Data from a preliminary study indicated a greater incidence of constipation among extremely low birth weight children. As more of these children are surviving, the awareness of constipation and related toileting problems in this population could lead to preventive intervention to ensure regular stooling (Cunningham, Taylor, Klein, Minich, & Hack, 2001).

Defecation disorders provide the pediatrician with the unique opportunity for anticipatory guidance and for the improvement of the health-related quality of life in patients and families. The first author's anecdotal experience has shown that children who have mastered this developmental task feel proud of themselves and that this sense of mastery is typically provides an intrinsic reward that is greater than any tangible reward or prize. In addition, once toilet training is achieved, parents often report an improvement in other behavioral issues. Research suggests that defecation disorders are being recognized at earlier ages, saving children and their families from unnecessary anguish, discomfort, and the potential for more serious long-standing problems (Fishman, Rappaport, Schonwald, & Norko, 2003). In addition, for the behavioral specialist, the opportunity to prevent psychological and behavioral sequelae from being added to medical problems that are very treatable is very rewarding.

APPENDIX A

STOOLING DIARY

Patients Name: _____

Date	Time	Amount of Stool (S, M, L)	Consistency (S, M, H)	Medication	Where Stooled

APPENDIX B

Annotated Bibliography

A. Children's Toileting books

1. *Uh, Oh Gotta Go!* – Bob McGrath
   A good book for toddlers which illustrates the process of toilet training from buying a potty to learning how to use it. Good illustrations.
2. *The Toddler's Potty Book* – Alida Allison
   This is a nice, simple story line for young children. The visuals are very good and toddlers react very positively.

3. *Max's Potty* – Harriet Ziefert
   This book is good for young toddlers. The flaps are interactive and fun for young children.
4. *Lift the Lid, Use the Potty* – Annie Ingle
   This book explains toilet training using a rabbit family. It is very good for young children because of all the flaps and lids. The younger kids like this book a lot. There is a cute example of a sticker chart that can be used at the end of the book.
5. *What Do You Do With A Potty?* – Marianne Borgardt
   This is a great pop-up book of what the potty is for. It is funny and "silly" and toddlers love this aspect. In addition, the pull-tabs and the flaps make it interactive and fun.
6. *The Princess and the Potty* – Wendy Cheyette Lewison
   This book is perfect for children with non-retentive fecal incontinence. It describes how important the concept of motivation for toilet training: the "moral" of the story is that the Princess has to decide for herself.
7. *I'm a Big Kid Now* –Joan Graham Brooks, M.D.
   This book is educational for parents. The boy/girl stories help parents know how to say things to children about toilet training in more detail. This aspect however, makes it wordy so that it is more appropriate for older toddlers.
8. *Going to the Potty* – Fred Rogers
   This book is highly recommended because of the realistic pictures of children in the bathroom and sitting on both potty chairs and toilets. Kids respond very well to this book.
9. *Everyone Poops* – Taro Gomi
   A classic with people all over the world, this book will bring smiles to children and adults. The message though, is important and presented in a clear "fun manner.
10. *It's Potty Time* – Smart Kids Publishing
    This book is a favorite with children of all ages because of the button that then produces the noise of a toilet flushing.
11. *Once Upon a Potty* – Alona Frankel
    This is a cute book, but it does not help children learn to recognize the urge to stool. It seems that it "just happens."

B. Books Related to Digestion

1. *What Happens to a Hamburger?* – Paul Showers
   This is an excellent book which describes the process of digestion in a kid friendly-manner. It is for older children. The illustrations are great.
2. *The Magic School Bus Inside the Human Body* – Joanne Cole
   This book is one of an excellent series which describes in a very kid-friendly way with great diagrams of what goes on inside the human body. The explanations in this book make it appropriate for older children.

APPENDIX C

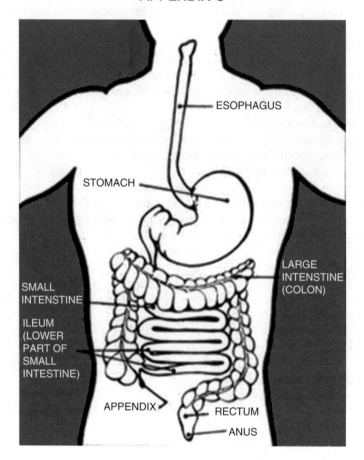

REFERENCES

Achenbach, T. M. (1991). *Manual of the Child Behavior Checklist 14–18 and 1991 Profile* (CBCL). Burlington, VT: University of Vermont. University Associates of Psychiatry.

American Psychiatric Association. (1994). *Diagnostic and statistical manual of mental disorders* (DSM-IV; 4th ed.). Washington, DC: American Psychiatric Association Press.

Arora, R., & Srinivasan, R. (2005). Is polyethylene glycol safe and effective for chronic constipation in children? *Archives of Disease in Children, 90*(6), 643–666.

Azrin, N. H., & Foxx, R. M. (1974). *Toilet training in less than a day*. New York: Simon and Schuster.

Benninga, M. A., Bueller, H. A., Heymana, H. A. S., Tzgat, G. N., & Taminieu, J. A. (1994). Is encopresis always the result of constipation? *Childhood, 71*, 186–193.

Benninga, M. A., & Taminieu, J. A. (2001). Diagnosis and treatment efficiency of functional non-retentive fecal soiling in childhood. *Journal of Pediatric Gastroenterology and Nutrition, 32*, S42–S43.

Benninga, M., Candy, D. C., Catto-Smith, A. G., Clayden, G., Loening-Baucke, V., Lorenzo, C. D., Nurko, S., Staiano, A. (2005). The Paris Consensus on Childhood Constipation

Terminology (PACCT) Group. *Journal of Pediatric Gastroenterology and Nutrition, 40*(3), 273–275.

Bishop. W. (2003). Infant dyschezia and functional constipation in infants and toddlers. *Archives of Pediatric and Adolescent Medicine, 157,* 661–664.

Blum, N. J. (1997). Behavioral characteristics of children with stool toileting refusal. *Pediatrics, 99,* 50–53.

Borowitz S. (2002). Treatment of childhood encopresis: A randomized trial comparing three treatment protocols. *Journal of Pediatric Nutrition, 34,* 378–384.

Brayden, R., & Altemeier, W. A. (1989). Encopresis and child sexual abuse. *Journal of the American Medical Association, 262*(17), 2446.

Broide, E., Pintov, S., Portnoy, S., Barg, J., Klinawski, E., Scapa, A. & (2001). Effectiveness of acupuncture for treatment of childhood constipation. *Digestive Diseases and Sciences, 46,* 1270–1275.

Brooks, R. C., Copen, R. M., Cox, D. J., Morris, J. Borowitz, S., & Setphen, J. (2000). Review of the treatment literature for encopresis, functional constipation, and stool-toileting refusal. *Annals of Behavioral Medicine, 22,* 260–267.

Chambless, D., Sanderson, W. C., Shoham, V., Johnson, S. B., Pope, K. S., Crits-Christoph, P., Baker, M., Johnson, B., Woods, S. R., Sue, S., Beutler, L., Williams, D. A., & McCurry, S. (1996). An update on empirically validated therapies. *Clinical Psychologist, 49,* 5–18.

Christophersen, E. R. (1991). Toileting problems in children. *Pediatric Annals, 20,* 241–244.

Clayden, G. S. (1992). Management of chronic constipation. *Archives of Disease in Children, 67,* 340–344.

Cox, D. J., Ritterband, L. M., Quillian, W., Kovatchev, B., Morris, J., Sutphen, J. et al. (2003). Assessment of behavioral mechanisms maintaining encopresis: Virginia Encopresis-Constipation Apperception Test. *Journal of Pediatric Psychology, 28*(6), 375–382.

Cunningham, C., Taylor, H. G., Klein, N., Minich, N., & Hack, M. (2001). Constipation among less than 750 gram birthweight children at 10 to 14 years of age. *Journal of Pediatric Gastroenterology and Nutrition, 33,* 23–29.

DiLorenzo, C. (1997). Chronic constipation and fecal incontinence in children with neurological and neuromuscular handicap. *Journal of Pediatric Gastroenterology and Nutrition, 25,* S37–S39.

Felt, B., Wise, C. G., Olson, A., Kochhar, P., Marcus, S., & Coran, A. (1999). Guideline for the management of pediatric idiopathic constipation and soiling. *Archives of Pediatric and Adolescent Medicine, 153,* 380–384.

Fishman, L., Rappaport, L., Cousineau, D., & Nurko, S. (2002). Early constipation and toilet training in children with encopresis. *Journal of Pediatric Gastroenterology and Nutrition, 34*(4), 385–388.

Fishman, L., Rappaport, L., Schonwald, A., & Nurko, S. (2003). Trends in referral to a single encopresis clinic over 20 years. *Pediatrics,* (5 pt. 1), 604–607.

Gershon, M. (1998). *The second brain.* New York: Columbia University Press.

Groves, J. A. (1982). Interdisciplinary treatment of encopresis in individuals with developmental disorders: Need and efficacy. *Monographs of the American Association of Mental Deficiency 1982*(5), 279–327.

Hatch, T. E. (1988). Encopresis and constipation in children. *Pediatric Clinics of North America, 35*(2), 257–280.

Howe, A. C., & Walker, C. E. (1992). Behavioral management of toilet training, enuresis, and encopresis. *Pediatric Clinics of North America, 39*(3), 413–432.

Hyams, J. S. (2000). Diet and gastrointestinal disease. *Current Opinion in Pediatrics, 14*(5), 567–569.

Hyman, P. E. (Ed.). (in press). *Childhood functional gastrointestinal disorders.* New York: Academy Professional Information Services.

Kuhn, B. R., Marcus, B. A., & Pitner, S. L. (1999). Treatment guidelines for primary nonretentive encopresis and stool toileting refusal. *American Family Physician, 59*(8), 2171–2178, 2184–2186.

Levine, M. D. (1975). Children with encopresis: A descriptive analysis. *Pediatrics 56*(3), 412–416.

Levine, M. D. (1981). The school child with encopresis. *Pediatric Review, 2,* 285–290.

Levine, M. D. (1982). Encopresis: Its potentiation, evaluation, and alleviation. *Pediatric Clinics of North America, 29,* 315–330.

Levine, M. D., & Bakow, H. (1976). Children with encopresis: A study of treatment outcome. *Pediatrics, 58*, 845–852.

Levy, J., & Volpert, D. (2004). Know the laxatives: A parent's guide to the successful management of functional constipation in infants and children. *International Foundation for Functional Gastrointestinal Disorders, 13*, 20–23.

Loening-Baucke, V. (1989). Factors determining outcome in children with chronic constipation and faecal soiling. *Gut, 30*, 999–1006.

Loening-Baucke, V. (1993). Constipation in early childhood: Patient characteristics, treatment, and long term follow up. *Gut, 34*, 1400–1404.

Loening-Baucke, V. (1995). Biofeedback treatment for chronic constipation and encopresis in childhood: Long-term outcome. *Pediatrics, 96*, 105–110.

Loening-Baucke, V. (2002). Polyethylene glycol without electrolytes for children with constipation and endocopresis. *Journal of Pediatric Gastroenterology and Nutrition, 34*, 372–377.

Luxem, M., & Christopherson, E. (1994). Behavioral toilet training in early childhood research, practice and implications. *Journal of Developmental and Behavioral Pediatrics, 15*, 370–378.

McClung, H. J., Boyne, L. I., & Heitlinger, L. (1995). Constipation and dietary fiber intake in children. *Pediatrics, 96*, 999–1001.

McClung, H. J., Boyne, L. I., Linshield, T., Heitlinger, L. A., Murray, R. D., Fyda, J., & Li, Bu (1993). Is combination therapy for encopresis nutritionally safe? *Pediatrics, 91*, 591–594.

McGinley, M. (2001). Management of encopresis and the parent's role. *NTPlus, 97*(20), 55–58.

McGrath, M. L., Mellon, M. W, & Murphy, L. (2000). Empirically supported treatment in pediatric psychology: Constipation and encopresis. *Journal of Pediatric Psychology, 25*, 225–254.

Mikkelsen, E. J. (2001). Enuresis and encopresis: ten years in progress. *Journal of the American Academy of Child and Adolescent Psychiatry, 40*, 1146–1158.

Nurko, S. Baker, S. S., Colletti, R. B., Croffie, J. M., DiLorenzo, C., Ector, W., & Liptak, G. S. (2001). Managing constipation: Evidence put to practice, *Contemporary Pediatrics, 18*, 56–66, 69.

Pashankar, D. S., Loening-Baucke, V., and Bishop, W. P. (2003). Safety of polyethylene glycol 3350 for the treatment of chronic constipation in children. *Archives of Pediatric and Adolescent Medicine, 157*(7), 661–664.

Rasquin-Weber, A., Hyman, P. E., Cucchiara, S., Fleisher, D. R., Hyams, J. S., Millar, P. J. & Staino, A. (1999). Childhood functional gastrointestinal disorders. *Gut, 45*(Suppl. II), II60–II68.

Rex, D. K., Fitzgerald, J. F., & Goulet, R. J. (1992). Chronic constipation with encopresis persisting beyond 15 years of age. *Diseases of the Colon Rectum, 35*, 242–244.

Ritterband, L., Cox, D., Walker, L., Kovatchev, B., McKnight, L., Patel, K. et al. (2003). An interest intervention as adjunctive therapy for pediatric encopresis. *Journal of Consulting and Clinical Psychology, 71*(5), 910–917.

Robin, G. (2000). Constipation in Children. *Clinical Evidence, 4,* 201–205.

Rockney, R. M., McQuade, W. H., Days, A. L., Linn, H. E., & Alario, A. J. (1996). Encopresis treatment outcome: Long term follow-up of 45 cases. *Journal of Developmental and Behavioral Pediatrics, 17*, 380–385.

Stark, L. J., Opipari, L.C., Donaldson, D. L. Danovsky, M. B., Rasile, D. A., & DelSanto, A. F. (1997). Evaluation of a standard protocol for retentive encopresis: A replication. *Journal of Pediatric Psychology, 22*(5), 619–633.

Stark, L. J., Spirito, A., Lewis, A. V., & Hart, K. J. (1990). Encopresis: Behavioral parameters associated with children who fail medical management. *Child Psychiatry and Human Development, 20*(3), 169–179.

Taubman, B. (1997). Toilet training and toileting refusal for stool only: A prospective study. *Pediatrics, 99*, 54–58.

van der Plas, R. N., Benninga, M. A., Buller, H. A., Bossuyt, P. M., Akkermans, L. M. A., & Taminiau, J. A. J. M. (1996). The additional effect of biofeedback training in the treatment of childhood constipation; a randomized controlled trial. *Lancet, 348*, 776–780.

van der Wal, M. F., Benninga, M. A., and Hirasing, R. A. (2005). The prevalence of encopresis in a multicultural population. *Journal of Pediatric Gastroenterological Nutrition, 40*(3), 345–348.

Vitito, L. (1999). Self-care interventions for the school-aged child with encopresis. *Gastro-enterology Nursing, 23*(2), 73–76.

Walker, C. E. (2002). Elimination disorders: Enuresis and encopresis. In M. Roberts (Ed.), *Handbook of pediatric psychology* (pp. 544–560). New York: Guilford.

Whitehead, W. E. (1992). Biofeedback treatment of gastrointestinal disorders. *Biofeedback and Self-Regulation, 17*(1), 59–76.

Whitehead, W. E., Parker, L. H., Masek, B. J., Caltaldo, M. F., & Freeman, J. M. (1981). Biofeedback treatment of fecal incompetence in patients with myelomeningocele. *Developmental Medicine and Child Neurology, 23*, 313–322.

Youssef, N. N., & DiLorenzo, C. (2001). The role of mobility in functional abdominal disorders in children. *Pediatric Annals, 30*, 24–30.

Case Studies: Treatment and Consultation Issues

INFLAMMATORY BOWEL DISEASE/CROHN'S DISEASE

Presenting Problem

Richard, a 16-year-old boy, was referred to me by his pediatric gastroen-terologist because of his difficulties related to his Crohn's disease (CD). His mother reported that Richard's mood appeared to be depressed, he was often teary, his activity level was low, and he was pessimistic about his future. Because of his embarrassment of having to frequently leave the class-room to use the bathroom, he refused to go to school and started home schooling.

History of Problem

Prior to his diagnosis at age 12, Richard had been a healthy child who was active in sports and an honor student. After the initial diagnosis of CD, he had a 3-and-a-half-year period of remission. At 16, despite consistency with the medical plan, his physical symptoms returned: Richard experi-enced significant cramping, he continued to lose weight, and he was pass-ing more than five loose stools a day. A colonoscopy indicated a flare-up of his Crohn's disease. He questioned, "Why did I have a flare-up now?" He was restarted on his prednisone and other medications. Embarrassment over bathroom-related issues and medication side effects such as cushingoid features led to school avoidance. At that time, the gastroenterologist referred him to me.

Cooperation from the school and the creation of a 504 plan for medical accommodations did not improve his anxiety regarding going to school. After a consultation with his gastroenterologist, a decision was made for him to be home schooled until he caught up with his schoolwork and his flare had subsided. Although home schooling decreased his anxiety about bathroom issues and he was able to get caught up in his schoolwork, Richard felt cut off from his friends and he had difficulty maintaining a schedule.

Richard became increasingly despondent as he realized he was still unable to manage his anxiety sufficiently to go to school. His parents who previously had differing opinions of how to manage his CD recognized that psychological factors were affecting his functioning as much as his CD.

I recommended consultation with a child psychiatrist who prescribed Prozac, which decreased his anxiety and his depressive symptoms.

Richard attended biweekly psychotherapy appointments and, in conjunction with consistency in his medical regimen, there was significant improvement in his physical and psychological condition. The gastroenterologist and I agreed that Richard would finish the school year at home, but that in the fall, he would return to school and that medical permission for a home tutor would not be provided.

Over the summer, he grew, he gained weight, and he was active with friends on the weekends. At the start of school he became anxious again. He admitted that he had stopped taking his Prozac during the summer because he had been "feeling so well." School avoidance was once again a problem: attempts to discuss and to plan for reentry to school was met with resistance, crying, and abdominal pain complaints. A repeat colonoscopy indicated that Richard's CD was in remission.

Developmental History

Richard's developmental history was unremarkable. He was the 7 lb. 6 oz. product of an uncomplicated pregnancy. His developmental milestones were within normal limits. He attended public high school where he was an excellent student. His teachers noted "his effort is outstanding" and that he "gets along well with the other students."

Richard lived with his mother and his older sister who was healthy. An older brother is in the army and he was also healthy. Family history is significant on the maternal side for irritable bowel syndrome (IBS). Richard's parents had been divorced eight years ago. Richard saw his father approximately once a week, but the relationship was strained.

Diagnostic Impression

Richard's high level of functioning was significantly impacted by his diagnosis of Crohn's disease. With the recurrence of his disease at 16, Richard began to exhibit anxiety, to the point of panic attacks in the morning prior to school. He became depressed when he could not participate in age-appropriate activities with his friends. Stress contributed to his heightened sensitivity to pain and to his cramping, which increased when he thought about having to use the bathrooms at school. Once this cycle began, Richard became overwhelmed and his anxiety became crippling.

Depressive symptoms included crying, anhedonia, and an increase in sleeping problems. Psychological diagnoses included (1) anxiety, with panic attacks prior to school, (2) dysthymia as a result of not being able to attend school and feelings of isolation, and (3) psychological factors affecting his physical condition.

Biopsychosocial Conceptualization

The positive family history of IBS on the maternal side indicates a physical predisposition to gastrointestinal (GI) problems. A sensitive, intelligent boy, he was acutely aware of calling attention to himself. Psychological stresses secondary to his illness included: having to frequently use the bathroom at school, the tension between his parents over the management of his school avoidance, and embarrassment due to medication side effects. Body image issues were of concern: Richard had not grown, he was very thin, and his cheeks were "moon-faced." Prior to school in the morning, he became anxious, which increased his intestinal cramping; consequently, his anxiety became more intense. Although Richard's anxiety did not cause his CD, it impacted his functioning in critical areas of his life: his heightened sensitivity to physical sensations contributed to his feelings of anxiety. His awareness of psychological issues increased his feelings of inadequacy and he became depressed. He started to view himself as a "sick person" who would not be able to function like his friends.

Treatment

Session 1

Richard presented as a thin, handsome 16-year-old boy who looked younger than his chronological age. His affect was flat and he became quite tearful when discussing missing his friends at school and feeling very lonely. He reported feeling increasing pressure from his father to attend school. His mother felt sorry for him and "because he's a good kid," she did not want to pressure him. His concerns regarding CD included the inability to predict the course of his illness and embarrassment and shame over bathroom-related issues. Richard completed the Childhood Depression Inventory. His scores indicated significant elevations in the following domains: negative mood, ineffectiveness, and anhedonia. His mother completed the Child Behavior Checklist (CBCL), and the results indicated significant elevations with respect to internalizing behaviors, particularly anxious/depressed mood and somatic complaints. His mother questioned, "Did stress cause his CD?"

In between the first two sessions I spoke with Richard's pediatric gastroenterologist and with the vice principal at his school to ensure that there was consistency among the health care providers and the school.

Sessions 2–5

A school reentry plan and a 504 plan were established. The school was very cooperative; Richard was to start back at school one hour a day and slowly increase his time there. The 504 plan, which documented his medical problem, specifically delineated accommodations for Richard that would help the management of his CD in the school setting. For example, Richard was able to use the nurse's bathroom, and if he were tired he could lay down for a period in her office. The first two days, Richard did well; he was happy to be at school, and he received a warm welcome from his friends. However, once the time increased to two classes, he started crying at home, reported that he was having cramps and that he "just couldn't go." He became panicky prior to school, and at our next visit, he sobbed that he "just didn't feel well." His parents pressured him and his father came to the house to take him, however, he still would not go to school.

Sessions 6–8

The goals of our biweekly sessions were: (1) to decrease anxiety and depressive symptoms, (2) to aid Richard in acceptance of his illness, and (3) to determine what activities he was capable of and what he was unable to do. The combination of taking Prozac, regular psychotherapy sessions, and being home schooled resulted in a decrease in Richard's anxiety. Acceptance of his illness was more difficult because of his anxiety, and he was not interested in meeting any other adolescents with CD. He was able to make use of the IBD library at the hospital, which is a collection of books and video tapes made by patients who wish to share their experiences in dealing with IBD. These materials helped in a nonthreatening manner to let Richard know the experiences of other adolescents with CD. As Richard started feeling better, he was more active and he began to recognize that his illness did not have to limit his functioning as much as it had.

   With good adherence to his medical regimen, Richard began to feel well physically. He stopped losing weight and he began having normal bowel movements 1 to 2 times a day.

Session 9

Richard was seen for a follow-up visit in the middle of the summer. He had gained weight and he had grown. He was active with his friends, riding his bike and playing basketball in his driveway. Anxiety symptoms had virtually disappeared and his mood was bright with no depressive symptoms. We discussed the proposed plan for school now only 6 weeks away and Richard reported that he "wanted to return." I spoke with the gastroenterologist and confirmed our plan for school reentry: a medical excuse would not be provided.

Sessions 10–12

Richard continued to gain weight and to grow; however, with the start of the school year, he began to have anxiety and some cramping returned. He questioned, "Will I be able to go away to college?" A repeat colonoscopy indicated his disease was still in remission. Richard acknowledged that he had been feeling so well that he had stopped taking his Prozac. The contract, which was reinforced by Richard's parents, his gastroenterologist, and myself, stipulated that he would not be given permission for home tutoring. Although he was very upset, he restarted the Prozac under his mother's supervision and progressive relaxation was introduced. He returned to school on an initially abbreviated schedule, which then was increased to a full day. He had difficulty at first, however, with a closely monitored schedule, reassurance, and support, his ability to stay in school improved.

Answers to Commonly Asked Questions

"Why did I have a flare-up now?"

The uncertainty of not being able to predict the course of IBD is one of the most difficult aspects of this disease. The realization that following the medical regimen, being careful with their diet, and going for follow-up visits to the gastroenterologist do not always prevent a recurrence is a source of anxiety for many children and adolescents. As in Richard's case, compliance with the medical treatment regimen did not prevent a flare-up from occurring 3-and-half years postdiagnosis.

"Is CD caused by psychological problems or stress?"

The exact etiology of CD is unknown. Current theories purport that psychological factors such as stress may exacerbate the illness, but they are not the primary cause. Psychological problems are more likely to be the *result* of the illness.

"Will I be able to go away to college?"

Concerns regarding independence and the ability to lead a "normal life" are concerns that become heightened because of CD. Most adolescents with CD do well, and the transitions to college and eventually adult gastroenterologists occur smoothly. However, each individual needs to be evaluated on a case-to-case basis.

GASTROESOPHAGEAL REFLUX DISEASE

Presenting Problem

Anna is a 9-year-old girl who presented with gastroesophageal reflux disease (GERD) and "worrying." Her parents reported that Anna was diagnosed with acid reflux, which they linked to stresses occurring at the start of the school year. They also reported that she was experiencing "anxiety as a result of the acid reflux." She worried when she felt ill and thought her symptoms were due to serious illnesses such as a heart attack or cancer. Anna described:

"I felt like my throat was closing up, like I can't breathe, my chest hurt and it scared me." Her pain and her worrying caused significant interference with her functioning. Anna did not want to attend school, she was in an irritable mood at home, and on weekends she did not want to participate in family outings, citing her pain and being tired as excuses.

History of Problem

According to her mother, Anna had always been an intense child and "a worrier." At the beginning of the school year (third grade), Anna began to complain frequently about the pain in her chest. A visit to the pediatrician determined that she had GERD. She was given a prescription for Zantac, which she took for a month and it decreased her reflux. Although there was improvement with her reflux, she continued to worry about somatic issues for herself and her family members. In addition, a number of stressors were identified: increased homework, girls teasing her, not being in the same class as her friends, and concerns about her grandparents' illnesses.

Developmental History

Anna was the result of an uncomplicated pregnancy resulting in a vaginal delivery. She had no neonatal problems. Developmental milestones were within normal limits. Early medical and social history was unremarkable. Anna lives with her parents, both of whom are Ph.D. scientists and are healthy. Her younger sister is healthy with no behavioral or medical problems. There have been no major stressors in the family, but the schedule for the children and parents is hectic: both parents work full time and the children participate in a number of activities. There is little "down time."

Assessment/Diagnostic Impression

Anna presents with GERD and anxiety. For Anna, the influence of these physical issues and psychological factors on each other was transactional.

Biopsychosocial Conceptualization

Paternal history of peptic ulcer disease (PUD) may represent a vulnerability to increased inflammation, leading to Anna's development of GERD. The social and academic stresses that Anna experienced were heightened because of her intense temperament, which in combination with a predisposition to inflammation contributed to her acid reflux. At the same time, her physical discomfort due to her acid reflux caused her to worry that her physical discomfort represented a serious illness, once again causing an increase in her anxiety.

Treatment

Session 1

I met with Anna's parents and I obtained a full medical and developmental history. They described a number of issues including her high level of worry, her sensitivity to somatic issues, and her problems socializing with other children at school. Her mother asked, *"Did stress cause her GERD?"* They completed the CBCL, which indicated significant elevations in internalizing behaviors, particularly anxiety and somatic concerns.

Session 2

Anna presented as a dark-haired intense 9-year-old girl. Her vocabulary was excellent, as was her ability to express her concerns, which included worries about her family's health, her sadness over the death of her cat, and her concerns when her chest hurt. She reported that this year was hard for her because she did not get along with the girls in her class. Her academic performance was not affected, but she often felt lonely and she was not invited to some birthday parties. Anna completed the Marsh Anxiety Scale for Children (MASC) and significant elevations were noted in the following domains: physical symptoms and social anxiety.

Session 3

We practiced progressive relaxation, making an audiotape of our practice for her to use at home. We discussed specific social skill strategies and we did some role playing of difficult situations that had arisen at school.

Sessions 4–6

We continued to review progressive relaxation techniques and added some visualization techniques. We discussed ongoing stresses at school and how to identify that the stress was bothering her. Anna practiced "listening to her body."

Session 7

Reviewed with parents the progress reported. Practical suggestions such as simplifying the family schedule, getting another cat, and inviting friends from school to the house were made. Her parents were praised for being proactive with inviting other children over to the house. Her parents questioned, *"How can we help her from feeling the normal stresses of life?"* We identified strategies that were helpful in decreasing stress, including: (1) keeping the daily schedule simple, (2) planning only one activity a day for weekends, and (3) discussing with Anna issues of concern to her immediately.

Sessions 8–10

Anna's progress with relaxation and visualization techniques was reviewed. We discussed Anna's ability to control her worries and reviewed each session how she was managing to deal with stresses. Anna asked, *"Will the GERD come back?"*

Answers to Commonly Asked Questions

"Did stress cause her GERD?"

Stress alone does not cause GERD. A multifactorial etiology including physiological vulnerability in combination with other factors is thought to be the cause. This issue needs to be reinforced with the patient and the family so that attribution of this illness is not seen as purely psychological.

"How can we help her from feeling stress?"

Stress exists. We cannot prevent feeling stress; however, the recognition and the management of stress can be improved so as to lessen its impact. Living with stress is something everyone needs to manage; however, for an intense highly intelligent child such as Anna, this was a challenge. Relaxation strategies can be preventative.

"Will her GERD reoccur?"

The recurrence of GERD cannot be predicted; however, improved recognition of symptoms may be helpful in alerting children earlier to a reoccurrence. In addition, stress management techniques, which often decrease the effect of stress, can have a preventative effect.

RECURRENT VOMITING/RUMINATION

Presenting Problem

Freddie is a 9-year-old, fourth grader, who presented with a 6-week history of recurrent vomiting. He vomited "whatever he just ate" after eating only two to five bites. The average amount of his emesis was roughly one quarter to one half cup. Liquids were worse than solids, with liquids coming up "fast and hard" soon after they went down.

History of Problem

Prior to the onset of vomiting, Freddie had coughed for 37 consecutive days. His cough began when he had an upper respiratory infection and never went away. Freddie's cough was eventually diagnosed as a "habit cough," and it ended the day he began vomiting. Throughout his coughing and vomiting, Freddie did not have any fever and lost minimal weight. His medical workup was negative. Over the 2 months prior to his psychological assessment, Freddie had gone to school only 2 days because of his physical difficulties, primarily his coughing. He had just returned to school, but his mother was taking him home for lunch so that his friends would not see him vomiting. Freddie's vomiting limited his peer activities and caused him to miss out on the sports he usually played. His parents had modified their lifestyles because of his problems (e.g., no eating at restaurants). Freddie was a good student who, despite missing a lot of school, had kept up with his classmates through tutoring. He was reportedly popular among other students. By his mother's report, Freddie was an emotionally sensitive boy who felt a great deal of self-imposed pressure to succeed. Freddie reported that he had no idea why he was vomiting. He perceived little control over his vomiting. Freddie's mother was adamant that his vomiting and coughing were not psychological or functional. At the same time, she began to ask herself, *"What did I do to cause these problems?"* She reported that upon learning of Freddie's psychological referral, Freddie's father blamed her for "babying" him too much.

Diagnostic Impression

Diagnostically, Freddie's recurrent vomiting or regurgitation is consistent with the rumination typically seen in children and adolescents of normal intelligence.

Biopsychosocial Conceptualization

In the absence of a physical or organic cause, Freddie's rumination, like his past coughing, was conceptualized as habitual in nature. Though he had no reason to vomit or regurgitate, especially after two to five bites, Freddie's vomiting occurred in almost automatic fashion. Though the mechanisms underlying ruminative behavior are varied, the vomiting or regurgitation often becomes habitual or conditioned, either physiologically or emotionally. Freddie's rumination was consistent with his history of habitual coughing and suggested a possible tendency toward habitual behaviors. For initial treatment planning, it was hypothesized that Freddie's ruminative behavior was maintained, in part, by the attention it elicited from his parents as well as any escape/avoidance it allowed from emotionally difficult situations. Given his emotionally sensitive nature, this latter function was reinforcing to Freddie.

Like Freddie's mother, many parents of children with functional GI disorders react strongly when the possibility of a psychological or functional disorder is raised. They interpret it as a suggestion that their child's problems are "all in the head" and react angrily and defensively. Many of these parents have suffered along with their children and are unable to accept this possibility. At the same time, they begin to question what role they may have had in the etiology of the child's difficulties. In their frustration, parents and other family members may begin to blame one another. As reflected in Freddie's father's response, poor or faulty childrearing is often implicated. For treatment to be effective, these maladaptive thoughts and reactions need to be addressed.

Treatment

Freddie's treatment was eight sessions in length. Much of the initial session was devoted to education. Freddie's recurrent vomiting or rumination was conceptualized as a habitual behavior, and possible maintaining factors were reviewed. Concerns about poor childrearing and blaming behaviors were discouraged, and parents were coached to focus on collaborative strategies to help Freddie break the habit of ruminating and gain self-control. The next two treatment sessions were devoted to teaching Freddie diaphragmatic breathing as well as various relaxation strategies, including progressive muscle relaxation and mental imagery. He was instructed to practice these techniques at home, and a behavioral contract was established to reward home practice sessions. In his next four sessions, Freddie practiced eating food without ruminating. He was trained to engage in brief relaxation strategies prior to eating and to use diaphragmatic breathing to counter urges to vomit. Freddie was also trained to use coping self-statements to handle negative thoughts and feelings while eating. Major treatment challenges included helping Freddie realize that he could eat more than several bites without ruminating and increasing his confidence in the use of diaphragmatic breathing as an effective self-control strategy. Over the same period, Freddie's parents were instructed to minimize their attention to his vomiting or regurgitation. Instead, they were to encourage and praise his practice of breathing and relaxation exercises and his efforts to eat without ruminating. Both parents were instructed to hold home practice sessions with Freddie, similar in nature to his office sessions. Involvement of both parents in this process was deemed essential for minimizing blaming and promoting a team effort at treatment. Though Freddie's parents were initially skeptical, they became increasingly engaged as he began to show slow but gradual progress. Over time, the parents became open to bigger lifestyle changes, such as letting Freddie eat lunch at school and going out to restaurants, in their effort to normalize his eating behavior. At a 6-week follow-up session, Freddie had improved to the point where he was no longer ruminating. He was eating lunch at school regularly without difficulties. Freddie was doing more with friends and showed interest in resuming his sports. His parents were relieved that he had progressed, and family functioning was much less stressed.

Answers to Commonly Asked Questions

"What did I do to cause these problems?"

As noted, many parents react strongly when the possibility of a functional GI disorder is raised. These parents expected a physical or organic cause for their child's symptoms to be identified, treated, and, at some point, cured. They are caught off-guard by the functional diagnosis and interpret it in maladaptive ways. Some are unable to accept the possibility that a functional disorder can cause so much distress and be so disruptive. Others interpret the diagnosis as a suggestion that their child is emotionally weak or behaviorally manipulative. They become angry at past providers who missed or mistreated the diagnosis. They may also become angry at their child for "allowing" his or her problems to get so far. Parents also begin to question the role they may have had in the etiology of their child's difficulties, including blaming one another in frustration.

It is critical to convey to parents that they are not to blame for their child's functional disorder. Although poor childrearing can add stress to a child's life as well as serve to maintain certain problem behaviors (e.g., parental sympathy reinforcing vomiting episodes), poor parenting alone does not cause the disorder. Presentation of a biopsychosocial conceptualization of the child's difficulties, itemizing hypothesized physical and psychological contributors, is important. Parental contributions should be discussed but not dwelt upon. Instead, the focus should be shifted to what parents can do to help their child manage symptoms more effectively and function more normally. Because much of the parental reaction to a functional diagnosis is felt to stem from uncertainty about what can be done, this shift in focus can be most empowering. Any blaming should be discouraged, and a joint parental effort to help the child should be promoted as the best means to a positive outcome.

RECURRENT ABDOMINAL PAIN

Presenting Problem

Ian is a 12-year, 3-month-old seventh grader, who presented with a several month history of intermittent abdominal pain. In the 3 days prior to his psychological assessment, Ian suffered continuous and severe abdominal pain. He reported that his pain was like "knives digging into (his) stomach." Ian had a tendency to become distressed and anxious at the onset of pain episodes. His emotionality worsened his pain and hindered his attempts to cope.

History of Problem

Ian had been previously diagnosed with gastroesophageal reflux despite a negative medical workup. He was tried on multiple reflux medications but showed little improvement. Prior to the onset of his pain problems, Ian did not exhibit significant emotional/behavioral difficulties. According to his mother, Ian had become increasingly irritable since the onset of pain. He was missing school and sitting out other usual activities. Ian identified multiple life stressors over the past 6 months. These included: (1) a difficult transition to middle school; (2) concerns about being overweight; (3) teasing by other students for being overly "brainy"; and (4) his mother's return to work for the first time since he had been born. Ian's family had been functioning well prior to his pain problems but was adversely affected by his difficulties. His parents were deeply concerned and gave him a great deal of attention because of his pain. Ian felt little control over his pain, and his parents were unsure of what they could do to help him.

Diagnostic Impression

Ian's symptom picture is consistent with Apley's original description of recurrent abdominal pain (RAP).

Biopsychosocial Conceptualization

Ian's case illustrates many of the characteristic features of childhood RAP. A previous medical diagnosis despite a negative workup and little improvement on medications is not uncommon in children with RAP and other functional GI disorders. This presentation leads parents to question whether the previous diagnosis was accurate or if it was given to satisfy or appease them. Questions about the appropriateness of past medications and what else can be done to help the child usually follow. In Ian's case, parents asked the following questions, *"How can you be sure that there is not a disease or something else going on?" "Should we have more tests done?" "What can we do to help Ian with his pain?"*

Though emotional difficulties may contribute to or trigger pain episodes, they may also be secondary to a child's pain. In Ian's case, the latter appeared true. As his pain persisted, Ian became more irritable. The stress and anxiety that Ian experienced at episode onset are also common. These may worsen a child's pain perceptions and negatively affect his or her coping efforts. When a child is unable to stay calm at the beginning of a pain episode, treatment must address this problem and provide the child with a self-regulation plan that assists with relaxation at the onset of pain.

The multiple stressors identified, especially those that were affecting Ian's day-to-day functioning, are common. The types of stressors that Ian identified—social stressors, self-esteem concerns, changes in daily living— are typical of those experienced by children Ian's age. The prominence of life stressors in the biopsychosocial model of functional GI disorders underscores the importance of stress in the etiology and maintenance of problems like RAP. It is important to note that life stress is often denied and the child's pain is identified as the only stressor in his or her life. Clearly, RAP is stressful and can have a major impact on the child and family. More often, however, stress is both a trigger for and consequence to the child's stomachaches. Assistance with how to cope with the stressful aspects of recurrent pains and managing life stress, in general, is frequently warranted.

As Ian's case illustrates, chronic, recurrent pain can be disruptive to family functioning. Often pain behaviors are inadvertently reinforced by parents' attempts to help their child. Unfortunately, parenting behaviors that are appropriate when caring for a child with acute pain are potentially counterproductive when the pain is chronic. Pain-associated disability is often seen and results when pain behaviors begin to serve positive functions for the child (e.g., increased parental attention, avoidance of negative school situations). For that reason, specific pain behavior management guidelines are important. Consistency between parents and collaboration between all parties involved (parents, teachers, health care professionals) is essential. To ensure success, all parties must buy in to and support the behavior management guidelines.

Treatment

Ian's treatment was six sessions in length, and a cognitive-behavioral systems approach served as its foundation. During the educational phase, special attention was given to an explanation of the process of diagnosing functional pain disorders. RAP was described in detail and distinguished from other possible causes for Ian's pain. This emphasis was important for allaying parental concerns about missing serious underlying conditions and assuring them of the appropriateness of Ian's diagnosis and proposed treatment plan. During the skills training phase, Ian was trained in self-regulation strategies to assist with pain coping and anxiety management. The latter focus was deemed essential for helping Ian stay calm at the onset of pain episodes. He identified diaphragmatic breathing and coping self-statements to be particularly useful in this regard. Specific pain behavior management strategies were recommended, with emphases on the promotion of normal daily activity and discouragement of pain behaviors. Because Ian's mother was unsure of how to respond when Ian felt "too sick" to attend school, his physician's input was solicited. Specific criteria were established (i.e., daily school attendance should be the norm; stay home only if there is fever, vomiting, or doctor's orders) and implemented on a consistent basis.

Improvement was evident almost from the beginning of treatment. Ian's ability to stay calm at the onset of pain improved dramatically and was a significant treatment milestone. Confident that he had nothing medically serious, his parents were consistently able to implement the recommended guidelines. Ian began to recognize that his parents were no longer responding to his pain as in the past. As he described, "They quit paying attention and ignored me when I complained about my stomachache so I quit moaning. I just tried to do something about it myself." At the conclusion of treatment, Ian reported minimal to no pain activity. The severity of his pain episodes had gone down significantly, and his parents reported almost no pain behaviors. He was attending school regularly again, and his home environment was beginning to normalize.

Answers to Commonly Asked Questions

"How can you be sure that there is not a disease or something else going on?"
We usually begin our response to this question by explaining that recurrent abdominal pain (RAP), or functional abdominal pain, is common. Almost 20% of children Ian's age experience RAP. It is important to convey that while there are over 100 organic causes of abdominal pain, a specific organic cause is found in only a small number of children. Serious, life-threatening physical causes are rare. A review of the typical assessment and diagnosis process, including routine lab tests, can be helpful. In discussing this process, note that there are usually "red flags" on history or examination that alert the clinician to physical explanations. Standard laboratory screening (e.g., complete blood count, erythrocyte sedimentation rate, stool studies, breath hydrogen testing) helps to rule out serious problems. Presentation of the Rome II criteria for childhood functional GI disorders can also be helpful. Since medical tests are not necessary or desirable for most of the functional disorders, these symptom-based criteria assist in making a positive diagnosis of a functional disorder (as opposed to one given after excluding all other possibilities). Finally, the Rule of Ones (Hyman, 1999) is useful to invoke. The Rule of Ones states that if a child has only one symptom, that symptom is probably functional. For example, abdominal pain alone is probably functional. Abdominal pain with fever or vomiting may not be functional and requires additional attention. Helping families overcome their concern that something else may be going on is critical to effective treatment and management. A sensitive and empathic, yet confident and reassuring manner is essential.

"Should we have more tests done?"
Typically, laboratory screening is limited. Again, since no medical test confirms a functional GI disorder, no tests are necessary. In rare cases, especially when a child is already scheduled and has been waiting for a long time, we will support completion of the scheduled testing. We do so, however, only with the agreement that after the test is done, no more testing will be scheduled and that the focus will be shifted toward treatment efforts.

"What can we do to help Ian with his pain?"
As noted in the chapter on RAP, there are numerous things that can be done to help Ian. These include symptom-based pharmacological therapies, dietary changes, cognitive-behavioral therapies, and alternative treatments. Parent management efforts should be directed toward encouraging normal activity and discouraging pain behavior.

FECAL INCONTINENCE DUE TO MEDICAL/BEHAVIORAL PROBLEMS

Presenting Problem

Brandon is a 3-and-a-half-year-old with Hirschsprung's disease who was referred to me by his surgeon for help in learning "how and when to stool." At the time of the referral, Brandon was impacted with soft fecal matter, but there were no medical reasons for impaction. His parents reported that they worried a lot and that they "sometimes teetered on the edge" of being "too into this poop thing" because of their anxiety.

History of Problem

Brandon's parents reported that he did not pass his meconium during his first 24 hours and he was throwing up "green stuff." He was sent to the ICU and discharged home, without a specific diagnosis. One week later, Brandon's parents brought him to the emergency room because he was "lifeless," "not eating," and "not stooling." He was hospitalized and a diagnosis of Hirschsprung's disease was made. His parents reported being "amazed and shocked" at a diagnosis that they had never even heard of. They questioned, *"Why us?"* During his admission, Brandon had surgery for a colostomy. At 6 months of age, he had another surgery; a duodenal pull through after which he began to stool from his rectum. Brandon did well until he was 1-and-a-half years old, when he developed a stricture in his small bowel and he had to have surgery to remove the scar tissue. Since the last surgery, he has had no further medical problems.

Developmental History

Brandon was the 7 lb. 10 oz. product of an unremarkable pregnancy resulting in an uncomplicated vaginal delivery. Despite significant medical issues, Brandon's developmental milestones were all within normal limits. Brandon lives with his parents and his 6-year-old brother who is healthy. Both parents work full time, but they have arranged their schedule so that one of them is always home with the children. The extended family is supportive, but extremely concerned.

Diagnostic Impression

Brandon presents with fecal incontinence due to his medical condition, Hirschsprung's disease. With the resolution of medical issues, behavioral management is essential to help Brandon learn how to use the toilet for stooling.

Biopsychosocial Conceptualization

Brandon's fecal incontinence resulting from his Hirschsprung's disease had a significant impact on him and his parents. Stooling was a complicated process for Brandon and he was hesitant to try using the toilet. Brandon's parents were very anxious about toilet training. They were concerned that he was becoming impacted regularly and because of the surgeon's recommendation they felt pressured to train him. They questioned, *"Can he be toilet trained?"* They recognized that not taking action was causing more medical intervention. However, they were not sure as to the approach or if he understood "what he needed to do." Both parents felt strongly "that he had been through a lot," consequently, following through with routines was difficult: if he put up any resistance, they relented.

Treatment

Prior to the first session, I spoke with the surgeon who reiterated that Brandon was now capable of stooling but he needed assistance in "learning how." The surgeon had recommended a bowel clean-out process, which his parents completed at home prior to our initial visit.

Session 1

I met with Brandon's parents and obtained a full medical and developmental history. They described their shock when the diagnosis was made since they and no one else in their families had ever heard of Hirschsprung's disease. His parents reported how frightening the surgeries had been for them; they acknowledged that they had worried about Brandon's possibly dying. Brandon's mother reported that while she intellectually recognized that the problem wasn't "her fault'" she still had a nagging sense of guilt, *"Did I do something wrong in my pregnancy to cause this?"*

Session 2

I met with Brandon and his father together. Goals included: (1) to help him relax, (2) to explain why he was coming to see me ("to learn to poop on the potty"), and (3) to determine his motivation and interest in toilet training. When I began talking about "pooping" he became quiet and looked at his father for reassurance, but he was cooperative and attentive.

We reviewed a very simple explanation of digestion and elimination, using GI charts and how it looks inside of him when the "poop gets stuck." We practiced blowing bubbles, while sitting on the toilet, to relax.

We practiced proper defecation dynamics: "how to strain." Brandon was to keep his hands on his stomach feeling the rectus abdominous muscles tighten as he took in a deep breath and pushed down, while keeping everything below his beltline relaxed. Reassurance that his body could "do this" and that it would not hurt was emphasized. Brandon was clearly interested in learning how to use the toilet, and I saw no evidence of oppositional behavior. A behavioral plan for both Brandon and his parents was created and implemented.

BRANDON'S PLAN

1. Practice sits on the toilet three times a day, approximately 15 to 20 minutes after meals for 6 to 8 minutes. He was to use bubbles to relax when first sitting.
2. Practice "how to strain" "the valsalva maneuver" when sitting. Stickers and a small piece of candy for a reward were given when he was successful.
3. Cleaning up his own pants should he have an episode of incontinence.
4. A special reward would be instituted such as playing a game with one of his parents should he spontaneously report that he has to use the toilet for stooling.

PARENTS' PLAN

1. Keep daily stooling diary.
2. Provide praise and encouragement, "You can do this," "Doesn't it feel good to be a big boy and do this yourself?"
3. Be consistent with rewards (e.g., sticker chart, candy, playing a game) and consequences (cleaning up his pants.)
4. Schedule regular follow-up visits, the first three to be scheduled weekly.

After this session, a letter was sent to Brandon's surgeon and his pediatrician, describing my initial visits and the proposed plan.

Sessions 3–8

During these weekly and then biweekly half-hour sessions, we began with a review of the behavioral plan and his sticker chart. Brandon, initially hesitant, was very cooperative with the plan. His body slowly adjusted to the schedule. Practicing the valsava maneuver and blowing bubbles, he relaxed and was able to stool, thus, gaining control over a process in which he previously had none. He was proud of himself.

His parents kept clear records of his stooling and they were consistent with the rewards and consequences. They understood the need for setting clear guidelines and they followed through with consequences. Accomplishing these specific tasks also contributed to a decrease in their anxiety.

Session 9

We reviewed the progress that had been made. His parents reported that information was helpful: "The more information you give us, the better, since we felt like you're alone and you don't know anyone else with this problem and you don't know what to expect. If you don't have information, you go to the Internet. The Internet is a great tool, but it's scary and it can make you worry needlessly." They also reported that they felt that the specific guidelines were set in place, so that if Brandon had any future problems, they felt they would know where to start. They questioned, *"Would this problem cause psychological 'scars'?"*

Answers to Commonly Asked Questions

"Why us?"

This is a common question that parents who have a child with a medical problem that seems to come "from nowhere" ask. Giving his parents a chance to express their feelings and reassuring them that Hirschsprung's is treatable helped Brandon's parents with the process of acceptance.

"Can he be toilet trained?"

My experience indicates that children with Hirschsprung's disease can be toilet trained. For Brandon, behavioral management with specific emphasis on teaching him how to strain was sufficient. Some children with Hirschsprung's disease will benefit from biofeedback, since studies document that external anal sphincter contraction in response to fecal distension is weak or absent in most children with Hirschsprung's disease.

"Did I do something wrong in my pregnancy to cause this?"

Parents, and mothers in particular, search for an answer as to why their child has an illness. Mothers often feel responsible and guilty even in light of information that contradicts their "feelings." The issue of feeling overly responsible needs to be addressed so that lingering guilt does not interfere with the implementation of the behavioral treatment plan.

"Would this leave psychological 'scars'?"

Parents understandably are worried about long-term psychological sequelae of the surgeries and the procedures. They were particularly concerned about issues related to toileting and that part of Brandon's body. We discussed the importance of their understanding their own anxiety so that it would not be transmitted to Brandon and of their answering Brandon's questions in a direct, matter-of-fact manner. They were encouraged not to be afraid to set limits and follow through with consequences.

RETENTIVE FECAL INCONTINENCE

Presenting Problem

Evan is a 7-year-old Caucasian boy referred to me by his pediatrician because of chronic constipation, stool retention, and frequent episodes of fecal incontinence. Evan typically had periods of 5 to 7 days when he would not stool. More days than not, there were smears of stool on his underpants.

When prompted by his parents to use the toilet, Evan would become angry and resistant and his parents were becoming increasingly frustrated.

History of Problem

Evan's problem with stool retention began when he was 2-and-a-half years of age. Prior to that time, he had been stooling on a regular basis without any difficulty or problems with constipation. His mother recalled that Evan had an "extremely hard stool, which was painful to pass." Stool retention became an increasing problem and a regimen of mineral oil, Milk of Magnesia, Senokot, and changes in his diet were implemented without improvement. At the age of 4, Evan became severely impacted. He was referred to a pediatric gastroenterologist. Enemas were added to his regimen on a monthly basis, yet no significant improvement was noted.

The family moved to the Cleveland area and Evan's new pediatrician, recognizing the problem, referred the family to a pediatric gastroenterologist who recommended a clean-out procedure and prescribed the use of Miralax 17 grams b.i.d. The clean-out procedure and the medication improved the problem of stool retention; however, episodes of fecal incontinence continued to occur both at home and at school. As the problem progressed, Evan was no longer able to stool without medication. Now in first grade, Evan was starting to be teased by the other children because "he smelled."

Developmental History

Evan's mother reported that he was the product of a full-term, uncomplicated pregnancy, delivered by Caesarian section. He was toilet trained for urine by age 3. Evan lives with his parents and his two siblings, both of whom are healthy. His father is a pastor at a local church and mother is a full-time homemaker. Family history is significant on the maternal side for stool retention as a child and chronic constipation. Evan's teacher reported that his academic performance has been good; however, he has "difficulty with his peers" and he is teased at school.

Diagnostic Impression

Evan presents with chronic constipation, stool retention, and fecal incontinence episodes, symptoms of retentive fecal incontinence (RFI). Hard stools due to constipation made defecation painful, and he started stool retention and the paradoxical contraction of his anal sphincter muscles.

Biopsychosocial Conceptualization

A maternal history of chronic constipation represents a physiological predisposition to a child's constipation. Psychosocial stresses contributed to the formation of this disorder, including the birth of a younger sibling coinciding with toilet training, the family's move to Ohio, his father's new job, and a decrease in support resulting from leaving a familiar environment and family members.

When Evan experienced the urge to have a bowel movement, because of pain due to hard bowel movements, there was the habitual paradoxical contraction of his external anal sphincter muscles. Practice sits on the toilet became times when stool retention would frequently occur. After sits, Evan would often have an episode of fecal incontinence because he would relax. At this point in time his parents asked another typical question, *"Is he doing this on purpose?"* They did not understand the process that was occurring and because of the close proximity in time, they believed that there was a volitional component to his incontinent episodes.

Evan's diagnosis of RFI was effecting his social development with respect to his self-care skills and his relationship with his peers and his parents. His parents were starting to view him as a child with "a psychological problem."

Treatment Plan

Session 1

The goals of the initial session were first, to obtain a full developmental and medical history, and second, to educate and to reassure Evan's parents that this is a common childhood disorder while also listening to their concerns. The final component of this parents' meeting included education about retentive fecal incontinence: its incidence and its etiology. The article by Jane Brody regarding this problem was given to them to read. In addition, information regarding how treatable this condition is was shared.

A common question came up during the initial evaluation, *"Is this problem the result of poor toilet training?"* Evan's mother, feeling increasingly guilty, was concerned that she had been too preoccupied with other issues, such as her new baby and the family's move, to focus on Evan's toileting. She questioned whether her own past problem with stool retention and constipation was responsible for "passing along this problem." Evan's father felt guilty that he had been overly concerned with what the members of his parish might think and consequently, he had been very strict with Evan.

In between the first two sessions, Evan's parents were instructed to follow the pediatric gastroenterologist's recommendations for a clean out. The importance of this step was stressed, as was the importance of consistency with the prescribed dosage of Miralax, 17 grams b.i.d.

Session 2

The goals of this session were to help Evan relax and to assess Evan's understanding of his problem. After his initial "shot" fears were relieved, Evan relaxed. He acknowledged that he did have problems with stooling and that he was "trying, but that sometimes I cannot feel when the poop is ready to come out." He also reported that some of the kids in his class teased him and that their comments made him "feel bad." Questions such as "Can you feel the poop coming out?" "Are you afraid that it will hurt coming out?" and "Some kids hold their poop inside because they're afraid it's going to hurt, did you ever do that?" were asked.

The next component in the treatment plan was to explain to Evan what was "happening in his body" so that we could work as "a team and fix it." A simple explanation of digestion and elimination was discussed using diagrams of the GI tract and supplementing them with pictures from a child's book for emphasis. The valsava maneuver was explained and practiced in the office to make sure Evan understood how to do it. Evan practiced straining in the office, while his mother placed her hands on his legs to feel if any tension was occurring, which would indicate paradoxical constriction. If she detected tension, she was to prompt Evan to relax.

A behavioral treatment plan was established for Evan and his parents.

EVAN'S PLAN

1. Taking his medicine.
2. Doing three practice sits a day for 8 to 10 minutes, one specifically after school.
3. Using the valsava technique while sitting. Evan was to be rewarded with a sticker for being compliant with each part of the plan. A certain number of stickers would earn him a prize.
4. If he had incontinent episodes, he needed to clean his pants himself.

Evan was able to repeat back the behavioral plan, indicating that he understood what was required.

PARENTS' PLAN

1. Keeping the stooling diary.
2. Following through with the established rewards and consequences.
3. Praising him for his effort and providing support and reassurance.

Sessions 3–8

Evan was seen for 6 half-hour follow-up visits during which his progress was monitored. These sessions focused on reinforcing the behavioral components of the plan and making sure that his parents were compliant with completing the stooling diary and giving the Miralax. At the first follow-up visit, Evan was doing well with taking his Miralax, but he was not cooperative with his practice sits. He would whine, argue, and protest when reminded to sit. He was commended for continuing to take his medication, however, consequences including no television or computer time were immediately instituted when he protested sitting.

Further visits indicated that the introduction of specific consequences was helpful in gaining Evan's cooperation. The consistent use of Miralax had produced soft-formed stools that made stooling easier. At this point his mother questioned, *"Will he become dependent on the Miralax?"*

The treatment component for Evan shifted from being reminded at specific times to sit on the toilet, to "listening to his body" and sitting. His parents were to reinforce this important step with comments such as "Aren't you proud that you are in charge now?" Rewards and consequences remained the same. Evan continued to make progress and he verbalized feeling "proud" about his "fixing" this problem.

Session 9

During the spring break from school, the family went to visit relatives for 2 weeks. It was a hectic time and both Evan and his parents had difficulty consistently following through with the treatment plan. Evan began to withhold his stool again since he was not on his regular schedule. His mother became very discouraged and she questioned, *"How long will this problem last?"* At home and with a follow-up visit to reinforce the "plans," Evan and his parents got "back on track."

Session 10

A follow-up visit 1 month later reviewed Evan's progress and made sure that any further questions were answered. The family was to follow-up with the pediatric gastroenterologist to decrease the Miralax dosage.

Answers to Commonly Asked Questions

"Is he doing this on purpose?"

Children with RFI often lose the sensation that they have to stool. The paradoxical contraction of the anal sphincter muscles becomes a habit due to the history of pain associated with hard stools. The toilet itself can become the trigger for this behavior and once off the toilet and relaxed, the child will stool, causing parents to believe that the child is doing it on purpose, but typically they are not.

"Is this problem a result of poor toilet training?"

Most parents of children with RFI believe that their poor parenting is the cause of this problem. Mothers in particular feel very guilty, and because this issue is not talked about they feel isolated and ashamed. Educating parents and clarifying the multifactorial etiology of RFI is an important and necessary step in treatment.

"Will he become dependent on the Miralax?"

Most children will be able to stop taking the Miralax after a period of soft stools occurring on a regular basis. Decreasing the dosage slowly seems to be most beneficial. In cases of severe chronic constipation, the pediatric gastroenterologist will evaluate dosages on a case-by-case basis.

"How long will this problem last?"

The response to this question is directly related to the level of compliance with the medical and behavioral plans. Our experience and the research literature indicate that most children do well. However, problems with severe chronic constipation may have to be monitored over time. Parents are encouraged to keep the stooling diary for *at least* 3 months posttreatment.

NONRETENTIVE FECAL INCONTINENCE

Presenting Problem

Michael is a 4-year-old boy who presents with a history of delayed stool toileting. His mother reported that he stools on a daily basis and that his stools are soft, but attempts to toilet train have not been successful. Michael will go behind a curtain in the family room and stool, he will not tell his parents, and it is only when his mother "smells something" and becomes upset will he go into the bathroom and with her help, clean himself up. His mother questioned, *"Why doesn't he want to be a 'big boy'?"* Michael's mother felt increasing pressure since entrance to preschool was contingent on his being toilet trained.

History of Problem

Toilet training began later with Michael because of a history of kidney infections. Michael saw a pediatric urologist and his kidney problem resolved with medication. Attempts at toilet training were not successful: neither bribery nor setting consequences worked. Because Michael's older brother had had a problem with retentive fecal incontinence, his mother was proactive in wanting to deal with this issue and she asked her pediatrician for a referral to a behavioral specialist.

Developmental History

Michael was the 7 lb. 7 oz. product of an uncomplicated pregnancy resulting in a vaginal delivery. His developmental milestones were within normal limits. He was toilet trained for urine at about 3 years of age. Michael lives with his parents and his two older brothers, both of whom are healthy.

Diagnostic Impression

Michael presents with nonretentive fecal incontinence. He stools on a daily basis without difficulty, his stools are soft and formed, and he does not report any pain with defecation. However, he is resistant to toilet training.

Biopsychosocial Conceptualization

Two factors impacted Michael's delayed toileting. The first was his kidney infections as a toddler, which delayed the timing of initiation of toilet training. The second was his older brother's problem with stool retention, which contributed to Michael's mother's hesitancy to "pressure" him for fear of the same situation reoccurring. Thus, when limits were established regarding toileting and he was resistant, she would become anxious and back down. Michael learned that he did not have to be compliant if he got upset.

Treatment Plan

Session 1

Michael's mother provided a full developmental and medical history. In addition, she described her attempts at toilet training and how the problem with her older son had affected her efforts with Michael. Although his mother recognized that she had not been consistent with Michael's training, she had lingering doubts and she questioned, *"Do you think there is a physical problem causing this?"*

Session 2

This session had three specific purposes: (1) to clarify with Michael why he was coming to see me ("to be a big boy like his brothers by using the potty"), (2) to establish the process of working together as a "team" using specific tasks that aid in reaching the mutually derived goal of being toilet trained for stool, and (3) to reassure him that other children had difficulty with this problem, but they learned how to do it.

Sessions 3–5

The most important component was to obtain Michael's cooperation so that the plan could succeed. A behavioral treatment plan based on the behavioral concepts of shaping and successive approximation was created, including the following steps in this process:

1. Michael was to get his own pull-up on when he stooled instead of asking his mother. He could stool in his familiar place.
2. He was then to move from behind the curtain and stool in his pull-up.
3. He was then to move to the edge of the family room and stool.
4. He was then to go into the bathroom and stool with his pull-up on.
5. He was to bend his knees slowly and them squat and stool with his pull-up on.
6. Michael was to sit on the toilet and stool with his pull-up on.

Michael was to try each step for 2 or 3 days. For every successful accomplishment, he received candy and a sticker kept on a large poster from his mother, and the choice of a Matchbox car from me. During this time period a book was made of pictures of Michael, and as he progressed through each step a new picture was added.

Sessions 6–7

Difficulty arose when we proceeded with the next step and cut a hole in the pull-up. Although cooperative, Michael was scared with this part of the plan and he began withholding his stool. His mother recognizing what was occurring because of issues with her older son and called the pediatrician who prescribed a half a cap of Miralax a day. In a few days, Michael began stooling again and he was cooperative with the plan. Behaviorally, he went back to sitting on the toilet with the diaper on and stooling daily.

Session 8

Michael sat on the toilet and stooled regularly for about 3 weeks, and at the end of this time, we asked if he wanted to try the hole or not using the pull-up, and he replied he wanted to try without the pull-up. Since he was scared, he practiced blowing bubbles to relax while sitting and we had him practice the valsalva technique, which, in combination of the use of the Miralax, he was able to stool easily. Michael was successful using the toilet without his pull-up after a few days. He was very proud of himself.

Answers to Commonly Asked Questions

"Why doesn't he want to be a 'big boy'?"
Michael's resistance to using the toilet for stooling may be the result of a number of factors: his initial urinary problems, his mother's hesitancy to set limits, his being the youngest child, and his brother's stool retention. Because all of Michael's other developmental milestones are within normal limits, it was likely that this issue would resolve. Sometimes "outside help" is necessary to change entrenched patterns.

"Do you think there is a physical problem causing this?"
Because of his urology problems, Michael's mother was hesitant to totally rule out a physical problem. Reviewing with her the pediatrician's diagnosis (nonretentive fecal incontinence), plus the fact that Michael had no difficulty in stool on a regular basis was helpful in reassuring her that this was a behavioral issue. Contact with the pediatrician had been important so that when stool retention occurred, it could be dealt with immediately. This concern faded in importance as Michael made progress with the behavioral plan.

SUMMARY

> I am convinced that the careful management of the mind is the concern
> of everyone and above all the physician, since it involves the health of the
> body. The mind has many powerful resources with which we may at times
> alleviate or cure diseases more surely or safely than with any other kind
> of remedy whatsoever. (Gaub in Rather, 1965, p. 195)

These lines by Gaub reiterate and summarize the emphasis we have placed on
the mind-body connection and a biopsychosocial perspective on pediatric GI
disorders. They also serve as a reminder that these notions are not new and,
in fact, have existed since long ago. The cases presented and discussed in this
final chapter illustrate a number of important lessons that we have learned
from our clinical experiences with children and adolescents with gastrointestinal disorders and their families. These lessons can be summarized by the
following points:

1. Familiarity with the physical symptoms, diagnostic procedures, and
   treatment modalities for common pediatric GI disorders is critical for
   fully understanding the patient's experience. It is important not to
   assume psychological etiologies for symptoms such as abdominal
   pain, weight loss, and fatigue.
2. The etiology of pediatric GI disorders is not dichotomous—physical
   etiology versus psychological origin. Even when physical causes have
   not been found, a psychological etiology cannot be assumed. It must
   be substantiated.
3. Diagnosis of a functional GI disorder does not mean that the problem is "all in the child's head" or psychologically caused. Nor does it
   mean that the child's parents are to blame.
4. By the time that many pediatric patients reach the specialist, their
   problematic behaviors (e.g., recurrent vomiting, stool withholding)
   have become habitual or conditioned. Symptom improvement and
   enhanced functioning require the acquisition of new, more adaptive
   habits or behaviors.
5. Treatment must acknowledge that the child is a dynamic "work in
   progress." Awareness of pertinent developmental issues can facilitate
   treatment and help to avoid clinical roadblocks.
6. Collaboration between the child, family, and clinician, along with
   other relevant parties (e.g., school staff) is often critical to the
   progress of treatment.
7. Our clinical experience is that children and families respond well to a
   biopsychosocial approach to treatment. Biopsychosocial treatment is
   clinically helpful, and the education and reassurance provided in this
   approach may have a preventive effect, both physically and psychologically.

Although the concept of a biopsychosocial approach may be accepted, its implementation is complicated by the restraints of our current medical care delivery system. Specifically, physicians are under increasing pressure to see more patients in a shorter period of time. Physicians and behavioral specialists may not be on the same insurance panels, thus the psychosocial intervention may not be covered by insurance. There are other practical issues that work against colloborative care, such as separate treatment locations and schedules that do not allow for convenient pairing of medical and behavioral appointments during the same time period.

Going forward, numerous questions about the nature of pediatric gastrointestinal disorders and their treatment remain. For example, which pediatric GI disorders may be precursors to adult GI disorders? In some conditions, such as IBD, is the childhood presentation a different disease from or just an earlier manifestation of the adult condition? What is the relative quality-of-life impact of pediatric GI disorders versus adult GI disorders? In terms of treatment, existing controlled research provides evidence that psychological/behavioral treatments, as a class of interventions, can be effective in reducing GI symptoms. Questions remain about the relative superiority of specific psychological treatments and the influence of active versus nonspecific aspects of these treatments (Lackner et al., 2004). Moreover, future investigations are needed to document the time- and cost-effectiveness of biopsychosocial approaches to pediatric GI disorders. Support or validation of these approaches has important implications for future efforts to care for pediatric GI disorders.

REFERENCES

Apley, J. H. (1959). *The child with abdominal pain.* London: Blackwell.

Brody, J. (1992). Silence on fecal incontinence is harmful: From 1 to 2 percent of children over 4 have the problem. *New York Times,* January 29, p. c3.

Hyman, J. S. (1999). Chronic and recurrent abdominal pain. In P. E. Hyman (Ed.) *Pediatric functional gastrointestinal disorders.* New York: Academic Professional Information Services.

Lackner, J. M., Mesmer, C., Morley, S., Dowzer, C., & Hamilton, S. (2004). Psychological treatements for irritable bowel syndrome: A systematic review and meta-analysis. *Journal of Consulting and Clinical Psychology, 72,* 1100–1113.

Rather, L. J. (1965). *Mind and body in eighteenth century medicine: A study based on Jerome Gaub De-Regime-mentis.* Berkeley: University of California Press.

Index